Hot Topics in Child and Adolescent Psychiatry

Editor

JUSTINE LARSON

CHILD AND ADOLESCENT PSYCHIATRIC CLINICS OF NORTH AMERICA

www.childpsych.theclinics.com

Consulting Editor
JUSTINE LARSON

January 2022 • Volume 31 • Number 1

ELSEVIER

1600 John F. Kennedy Boulevard • Suite 1800 • Philadelphia, Pennsylvania, 19103-2899

http://www.theclinics.com

CHILD AND ADOLESCENT PSYCHIATRIC CLINICS OF NORTH AMERICA Volume 31, Number 1
January 2022 ISSN 1056–4993, ISBN-13: 978-0-323-91969-2

Editor: Lauren Boyle
Developmental Editor: Arlene Campos

Child and Adolescent Psychiatric Clinics of North America (ISSN 1056-4993) is published quarterly by Elsevier Inc., 360 Park Avenue South, New York, NY 10010-1710. Months of issue are January, April, July, and October. Business and Editorial Offices: 1600 John F. Kennedy Boulevard, Suite 1800, Philadelphia, PA 19103-2899. Periodicals postage paid at New York, NY and additional mailing offices. Subscription prices are $358.00 per year (US individuals), $869.00 per year (US institutions), $100.00 per year (US & Canadian students), $399.00 per year (Canadian individuals), $895.00 per year (Canadian institutions), $459.00 per year (international individuals), $895.00 per year (international institutions), and $200.00 per year (international students). International air speed delivery is included in all *Clinics* subscription prices. All prices are subject to change without notice. **POSTMASTER:** Send address changes to *Child and Adolescent Psychiatric Clinics of North America*, Elsevier Health Sciences Division, Subscription Customer Service, 3251 Riverport Lane, Maryland Heights, MO 63043. **Customer Service: 1-800-654-2452 (U.S. and Canada); 314-447-8871 (outside U.S. and Canada). Fax: 314-447-8029. E-mail:** JournalsCustomer Service-usa@elsevier.com **(for print support) or** journalsonlinesupport-usa@elsevier.com **(for online support).**

Reprints. For copies of 100 or more of articles in this publication, please contact the Commercial Reprints Department, Elsevier Inc., 360 Park Avenue South, New York, New York 10010-1710 Tel.: 212-633-3874; Fax: 212-633-3820, E-mail: reprints@elsevier.com.

Child and Adolescent Psychiatric Clinics of North America is covered in *MEDLINE/PubMed (Index Medicus), ISI, SSCI, Research Alert, Social Search, Current Contents,* and *EMBASE/Excerpta Medica.*

Contributors

CONSULTING EDITOR

JUSTINE LARSON, MD, MPH, DFAACAP
Medical Director, Schools and Residential Treatment, Consulting Editor, Child and Adolescent Psychiatric Clinics of North America, Sheppard Pratt , Rockville, Maryland, USA

EDITOR

JUSTINE LARSON, MD, MPH, DFAACAP
Medical Director, Schools and Residential Treatment, Consulting Editor, Child and Adolescent Psychiatric Clinics of North America, Sheppard Pratt , Rockville, Maryland, USA

AUTHORS

MERLIN ARIEFDJOHAN, PhD, MPH
Department of Psychiatry, University of Colorado Anschutz Medical Campus, Aurora, Colorado, USA

CHRISTINA D. BETHELL, PhD, MBA, MPH
Professor, Department of Population, Family and Reproductive Health, Johns Hopkins Bloomberg School of Public Health, Baltimore, Maryland, USA

COURTNEY BLACKWELL, PhD
Research Assistant Scientist, Department of Medical Social Sciences, Northwestern University Feinberg School of Medicine, Chicago, Illinois, USA

JEANNE FUNK BROCKMYER, PhD
Distinguished University Professor Emerita, Department of Psychology, University of Toledo, Toledo, Ohio, USA

JUDITH A. COHEN, MD
Professor of Psychiatry, Allegheny Health Network, Drexel University College of Medicine, Pittsburgh, Pennsylvania, USA

RACHAEL A. CROFFORD, MS
College of Education and Health Professions, University of Arkansas, Fayetteville, Arkansas, USA

MOLLY DAFFNER-DEMING, PhD
Department of Education and Human Services, Lehigh University, Bethlehem, Pennsylvania, USA

AMANDA DOWNEY, MD, FAAP
Assistant Professor of Pediatrics and Psychiatry, Division of Adolescent and Young Adult Medicine, Department of Pediatrics, Department of Psychiatry and Behavioral Sciences University of California, San Francisco, San Francisco, California, USA

GEORGE J. DUPAUL, PhD
Department of Education and Human Services, Lehigh University, Bethlehem, Pennsylvania, USA

YAEL DVIR, MD
Associate Professor of Psychiatry and Pediatrics, Department of Psychiatry, University of Massachusetts Chan Medical School, Worcester, Massachusetts, USA

CÉSAR G. ESCOBAR-VIERA, MD, PhD
Department of Psychiatry, University of Pittsburgh School of Medicine, Pittsburgh, Pennsylvania, USA

SANDRA L. FRITSCH, MD, MSEd
Pediatric Mental Health Institute, Children's Hospital Colorado, Department of Psychiatry, University of Colorado Anschutz Medical Campus, Aurora, Colorado, USA

ANDREW S. GARNER, MD, PhD
Clinical Professor, Case Western Reserve University School of Medicine, Cleveland, Ohio, USA

JENNA GLOVER, PhD
Pediatric Mental Health Institute, Children's Hospital Colorado, Department of Psychiatry, University of Colorado Anschutz Medical Campus, Aurora, Colorado, USA

NARANGEREL GOMBOJAV, MD, PhD
Assistant Scientist, Department of Population, Family and Reproductive Health, Johns Hopkins Bloomberg School of Public Health, Baltimore, Maryland, USA

MATTHEW J. GORMLEY, PhD
Department of Education and Human Services, Lehigh University, Bethlehem, Pennsylvania, USA; University of Nebraska-Lincoln, Lincoln, Nebraska, USA

DAVID N. GREENFIELD, PhD, MS, ABPP
Founder and Medical Director, The Center for Internet and Technology Addiction, West Hartford, Connecticut, USA; Consulting Medical Director, Greenfield Pathway for Video Game and Technology Addiction @ Lifeskills South Florida; University of Connecticut, School of Medicine, Department of Psychiatry (former), Farmington, Connecticut, USA

LAURENCE HELLER, PhD
Director, NeuroAffective Relational Model Training Institute, Inc, Littleton, Colorado, USA

ANTHONY P. MANNARINO, PhD
Vice Chair and Professor, Psychiatry and Behavioral Health Institute, Allegheny Health Network, Drexel University College of Medicine, Pittsburgh, Pennsylvania, USA

TAMAR MENDELSON, PhD
Professor, Department of Population, Family and Reproductive Health, Johns Hopkins Bloomberg School of Public Health, Baltimore, Maryland, USA

SARA PAWLOWSKI, MD
Child and Adolescent Psychiatry, University of Vermont Medical Center, Burlington, Vermont, USA

KRISTI L. PERRYMAN, PhD
College of Education and Health Professions, University of Arkansas, Fayetteville, Arkansas, USA

BRIAN A. PRIMACK, MD, PhD
College of Education and Health Professions, University of Arkansas, Fayetteville, Arkansas, USA

DAVID C. RETTEW, MD
Child and Adolescent Psychiatry, University of Vermont Medical Center, Burlington, Vermont, USA

RACHEL F. RODGERS, PhD
Department of Applied Psychology, APPEAR, Northeastern University, Boston, Massachusetts, USA; Department of Psychiatric Emergency and Acute Care, Lapeyronie Hospital, CHRU Montpellier, France

JOHN S. ROZEL, MD, MSL, DFAPA
Associate Professor of Psychiatry & Adjunct Professor of Law, University of Pittsburgh, Medical Director, resolve Crisis Services of UPMC Western Psychiatric Hospital Pittsburgh, Pennsylvania, USA

JENNA SAUL, MD
Rogers Behavioral Health, Oconomowoc, Wisconsin, USA; Child and Adolescent Psychiatry Consulting, Marshfield, Wisconsin, USA

McKENNA SAUL
University of Wisconsin, Parkside, Kenosha, Wisconsin, USA

CAMILLE TASTENHOYE, MD
Child and Adolescent Psychiatry Fellow, PGY4, Department of Psychiatry, University of Pittsburgh School of Medicine, UPMC Western Psychiatric Hospital, Pittsburgh, Pennsylvania, USA

KEVIN WHITLEY, MD, MA
Attending Psychiatrist, Southwood Psychiatric Hospital, Pittsburgh, Pennsylvania, USA

Contents

Bullying is a complex and widespread public health issue that affects chil-dren of all ages and adults. For decades, childhood bullying has been viewed as an unpleasant but generally harmless rite of passage that carries with it few long-term consequences. Research has increasingly documented the serious and long-term behavioral and health conse-quences of bullying. This article addresses several features of bullying including epidemiology, psychological and physical impact, and the role of health care providers in bullying detection, intervention, and prevention.

Social media (SM) use is prevalent among youth, who are at critical junc-tures around developmental tasks such as identity development and establishment of social norms. In the United States, approximately 84% of young adults ages 18-29 use SM, and about 95% of youth ages 13-17 own smartphones, and nearly all of them use SM. The purpose of this review is to broadly summarize research that has explored how SM in-terfaces with psychosocial development and mental health conditions as of May 2021. We also aimed to summarize important directions for future research. Emerging data related to the COVID-19 were included.

Mental health treatment of juvenile offenders and undocumented immi-grant youth in detention provides a unique opportunity for treatment pro-viders. Although the work may be challenging, the clinical needs and opportunities for early and meaningful interventions are significant. One of the best clinical experiences a psychiatrist can have is working with extremely high-risk youth to help them find safer and better developmental pathways. Few settings can offer such an opportunity to leverage clinical skills to improve the lives and futures of children and adolescents as are afforded to those professionals lucky enough to work in juvenile justice settings.

Nearly 70% (67.6%) of US children with mental, emotional, and behavioral problems (MEB) experienced significant social health risks (SHR) and/or relational health risks (RHR). Shifts are needed in child mental health promotion, prevention, diagnosis, and treatment to address both RHR and SHR. Public health approaches are needed that engage families, youth, and the range of child-serving professionals in collaborative efforts to prevent and mitigate RHR and SHR and promote positive mental health at a community level. Building strong family resilience and connection may improve SR and, in turn, academic and social outcomes among all US children with or without MEB.

This article discusses child onset anxiety disorders in conjunction with the risks and benefits of the rapidly changing digital world including screen time, social media, and potential treatment platforms. A section includes the impact of pandemic stressors including social distancing, quarantining, the association of the pandemic and youth mental health, and prolonged screen time.

Significant evidence suggests strong links between childhood trauma and psychosis, with childhood trauma considered a significant risk factor for psychosis, causing a more severe presentation of psychotic illness with a dose-response effect. The relationship between anxiety, mood, post-traumatic stress disorder, and childhood trauma and psychosis and the difficulties distinguishing between overlapping symptoms require careful attention of the treating clinician considering the presentation and treatment course. Finally, there also appears to be a link between childhood trauma and violent behavior in individuals with psychotic illness. More research is needed into the effectiveness and safety of trauma-focused psychotherapeutic interventions.

Common addictive patterns found specifically with Internet screen use often present with similar symptomatology to other behavioral and substance-based addictions, although severity and impairment vary widely. And there are numerous specific characteristics which appear to contribute to the addictive properties of Internet behavior. This article addresses clinical treatment strategies applicable to Internet and video game addiction (IVGA). It also presets working definitions for the addictive use of the Internet and identifies the unique behavioral aspects of Internet and screen use disorders. This article also reviews the etiologic and neurobiological antecedents to Internet and video game addiction, provides samples of the relevant treatment literature, and presents the CITA model of treatment.

Jeanne Funk Brockmyer

Desensitization, the reduction of cognitive, emotional, and/or behavioral responses to a stimulus, is an automatic and unconscious phenomenon often experienced in everyday life. Exposure to violent media, especially violent video games, may cause desensitization to real-life violence. Desensitization to violence blocks empathy which is needed to trigger the moral reasoning process that triggers prosocial responding. Representative research was reviewed to examine links between exposure to violent video games and desensitization to violence in children and adolescents. It was concluded that exposure to violent video games increases the risk of desensitization to violence, which in turn may increase aggression and decrease prosocial behavior. Parents should be counseled to discuss the differences between real and screen violence, to encourage nonviolent problem-solving, and to provide empathy-building experiences for their children.

Judith A. Cohen and Anthony P. Mannarino

Child trauma is a serious societal problem. At least one trauma is reported by two-thirds of American children and adolescents Despite children's inherent resilience, trauma exposure is associated with increased risk for medical and mental health problems including posttraumatic stress disorder, depression, anxiety, substance abuse, and attempted and completed suicide. Early identification and treatment of traumatized children can prevent these potentially serious and long-term negative outcomes.

George J. DuPaul, Matthew J. Gormley, and Molly Daffner-Deming

Children with attention-deficit/hyperactivity disorder experience significant academic, social, and behavioral impairments in elementary school settings. Although psychopharmacologic treatments can improve symptomatic behaviors, these rarely are sufficient for enhancing school performance. Thus, medication should be supplemented by one or more school interventions, including behavioral strategies, academic interventions, behavioral peer interventions, organizational skills training, and self-regulation strategies. Although all of these school interventions have been found effective, classroom behavioral strategies, organizational skills training, and self-regulation strategies have the strongest empirical support. Clinicians should collaborate with school mental health professionals to encourage implementation of effective school interventions across school years.

The role of traditional media (television and magazines) in creating eating disorder risk has long been a topic of discussion and research, but the proliferation of social media and rapid increase in the use of the Internet by adolescents generates new dynamics and new risks for the development and maintenance of eating disorders. Recent research describes the relationship between Internet and social media use and eating disorders risk, with the greatest associations found among youth with high levels of engagement and investment in photo-based activities and platforms. Here, we review different types of online content and how they are relevant to eating disorders and consider the theoretical frameworks predicting relationships between Internet and social media and eating disorders, before examining the empirical evidence for the risks posed by the online content in the development and maintenance of eating disorders. We describe proeating disorder content specifically and examine the research related to it; we then consider the implications of such content, highlight directions for future research, and discuss possible prevention and intervention strategies.

CHILD AND ADOLESCENT PSYCHIATRIC CLINICS

FORTHCOMING ISSUES

APRIL 2022
Addressing Systemic Racism and Disparate Mental Health Outcomes for Youth of Color
Lisa Fortuna, Cheryl S. Al-Mateen, Lisa Cullins, and David Lohr, *Editors*

JULY 2022
Updates in Pharmacologic Strategies in ADHD
Jeffrey H. Newcorn, and Timothy E. Wilens, *Editors*

JANUARY 2022
Adolescent Cannabis Use
Paula Riggs, Jesse D. Hinckley, and J. Megan Ross, *Editors*

RECENT ISSUES

OCTOBER 2021
Collaborative Partnerships to Advance Practice
Suzie Nelson, Jessica Jeffrey, and Mark Borer, *Editors*

JULY 2021
Emotion Dysregulation and Outbursts in Children and Adolescents: Part II
Manpreet K. Singh, Gabrielle A. Carlson, *Editors*

APRIL 2021
Emotion Dysregulation and Outbursts in Children and Adolescents: Part I
Gabrielle A. Carlson, Manpreet K. Singh, Editors, *Editors*

SERIES OF RELATED INTEREST
Psychiatric Clinics of North America
https://www.psych.theclinics.com/
Pediatric Clinics of North America
https://www.pediatric.theclinics.com/
Neurologic Clinics
https://www.neurologic.theclinics.com/

THE CLINICS ARE AVAILABLE ONLINE!
Access your subscription at:
www.theclinics.com

CHILD AND ADOLESCENT PSYCHIATRIC CLINICS

Preface
Hot Topics

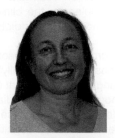

Justine Larson, MD, MPH, MHS
Editor

As the new Consulting Editor for the *Child and Adolescent Psychiatric Clinics of North America*, I am pleased to act as the Guest Editor for this "Hot Topics" issue. This issue is an assortment of updated articles that are the most downloaded articles in the past decade, a sort of "Greatest Hits" from the *Child and Adolescent Psychiatric Clinics of North America*. One may be able to glean some interesting information about what clinicians are downloading, perhaps it reveals something about gaps in the field, areas of interest, and areas in which clinicians feel that need to learn more.

In examining the different "Hot Topics" articles, several themes emerge: social media and electronics; trauma and interpersonal conflict; and the contexts in which children and adolescents live.

Social media and electronics are increasingly important in the lives of the vast majority of children and adolescents, but even more so during the current pandemic. Families look to clinicians on how to best support their children's use of electronics and on the Internet. As social media and electronic use increase among children and adolescents, there are important questions that arise for both clinicians and families: How much electronic use is too much? Are video games harmful? How does social media and the Internet use impact the mental health of children and adolescents? In "Social media as it interfaces with psychosocial development and mental illness in transitional age youth," the authors note increasing levels of use among adolescents in the past decade, and they review the recent literature examining associations between social media use and symptoms of anxiety and depression. The article, "#kids anxiety and the digital world," further explores the impact of social media on anxiety, again finding an association between use and higher levels of anxiety. The authors also note a potential positive role of the Internet and social media for children and adolescents at risk for or living with anxiety. "Adolescent eating disorder risk and the online world" examines the role of the Internet and social media on eating disorder symptoms, describing the scientific literature and reporting a positive association with

Child Adolesc Psychiatric Clin N Am 31 (2022) xiii–xv
https://doi.org/10.1016/j.chc.2021.09.005
1056-4993/22/© 2021 Published by Elsevier Inc.

childpsych.theclinics.com

increasing use and eating disorder symptoms, particularly with photo-based platforms. In "Playing violent video games and desensitization to violence," the author describes the phenomenon of desensitization, defined as a reduction of cognitive, emotional, and/or behavioral responses to a stimulus, and explores the scientific literature supporting a link between violent video games and desensitization to real-life violence. "Clinical considerations in Internet and video game addiction treatment" offers some nut-and-bolts pearls about how to address this problem in the clinical setting and discusses the commonalities between Internet and video game addiction and other substance use disorders.

Another common thread in the articles is in the area of trauma and interpersonal conflict. The article "Bullying" summarizes the mental health consequences of bullying and describes several strategies to address and prevent bullying when working at the individual and community level. "Childhood trauma and psychosis" explores the diagnostic links between psychosis and trauma, examining in depth a specific case of cooccurring posttraumatic stress disorder and psychosis. "Trauma-focused cognitive behavior therapy for traumatized children and families" provides an excellent description of the components of trauma-focused cognitive behavior therapy and summarizes some of the nuances and outcomes of this treatment.

A third theme among this collection of articles could be the contexts in which children and adolescents live and learn, and how these contexts can be deleterious or helpful. "Social and relational health risks and common mental health problems among US children: the mitigating role of family resilience and connection to promote positive socioemotional and school-related outcomes" describes a study utilizing a creative methodology to examine the correlation of mental health problems and social and relational health risks. The authors found that the prevalence of common mental, emotional, and behavioral conditions among US children varied 4-fold according to the number of relational health risks and/or social health risks they experience. The study further supports the notion that many child and adolescent psychiatrists know well from clinical experience: that family and community contexts matter for the mental health of children and adolescents. Last, "School-based interventions for elementary school students with attention-deficit/hyperactivity disorder" provides an overview of the evidence of approaches to children with attention-deficit/hyperactivity disorder in elementary schools, dividing the interventions into behavioral strategies, academic interventions, behavioral peer interventions, organizational skills training, and self-regulation strategies. It is encouraging that these interventions have been found to be effective, and that the strongest evidence exists for classroom behavioral strategies, organizational skills training, and self-regulation strategies.

The common themes among these articles: electronic use, trauma, and children's contexts, are particularly salient at this time, as we continue to struggle with the pandemic and natural disasters. I am looking forward to my term as the Consulting Editor and am excited about timely and interesting issues of the *Child and Adolescent Psychiatric Clinics of North America* on the horizon. I hope that they can offer clinicians knowledge and tools to provide care during these unprecedented times.

Justine Larson, MD, MPH, MHS
Schools and Residential Treatment
Sheppard Pratt
Baltimore, MD 21204, USA

E-mail address:
Justine.Larson1@sheppardpratt.org

Bullying: An Update

David C. Rettew, MD, Sara Pawlowski, MD*

KEYWORDS

- Bullying • Prevention • Adverse child experience • Peer aggression

KEY POINTS

- Bullying refers to repetitive and intentional peer aggression where there exists a power imbalance.
- Research has increasingly documented the serious and long-term behavioral and health consequences of bullying.
- Several strategies have demonstrated efficacy in addressing and preventing bullying on the individual level and more broadly within schools and communities.

INTRODUCTION

This article represents an updated version of the authors' original article from 2018.[1] Bullying is a complex and widespread public health issue that affects children of all ages and adults. For decades, childhood bullying has been viewed as an unpleasant but generally harmless rite of passage that carries with it few long-term consequences. Portrayals of bullying in countless books and movies depict bully-victims as inevitably resilient and victorious, whereas the bully eventually meets with justice. In the real world, however, such an optimistic view has been tempered by many high-profile suicides coupled with an accumulating literature that has revealed, to the surprise of many, how serious and widespread the sequelae of bullying can be. Current thinking now reflects an understanding of bullying less as an inevitable component of growing up and more as a form of trauma with long-term serious physical and psychological consequences for bullies, victims, and those who oscillate between both roles (bully-victims). With this increased concern about bullying has fortunately come a surge of research directed at advancing basic understanding of bullying behavior and at guiding antibullying interventions on the individual and community level. The following sections address several features of bullying including epidemiology, psychological and physical impact, and the role of health care providers in bullying detection, intervention, and prevention.

Child & Adolescent Psychiatry, University of Vermont Medical Center, 1 South Prospect Street, Arnold 3, Burlington, VT 05401, USA
* Corresponding author. .
E-mail address: sara.pawlowski@uvmhealth.org

Child Adolesc Psychiatric Clin N Am 31 (2022) 1–9
https://doi.org/10.1016/j.chc.2021.09.001
1056-4993/22/© 2021 Published by Elsevier Inc.
childpsych.theclinics.com

DEFINITION AND PHENOMENOLOGY OF BULLYING

Bullying is often defined as repetitive and intentional aggressive behavior by one individual or group against another in situations where there exists some sort of power differential between the bully and the victim in terms of physical size, social status, or other features.[2] Bullying behavior can include anything from name-calling to outright physical assault. What has been termed relational bullying can involve actions that can occur between friends and acquaintances such as spreading rumors or the active ignoring or exclusion of certain individuals.

Of particular interest lately is cyberbullying, which involves harassing and demeaning text messages, emails, and social media posts. Following the writing of the authors' original article, the landscape of social media has expanded with the arrival of more apps with unprecedented capabilities for communication and connection. With this emergence has also come more potential cyberbullying opportunities and vulnerabilities. Per the Pew Research Institute, "the likelihood of teens facing abusive behavior varies by how often teens go online" with particular concern for "constant users." The duration of time online correlates with an increased risk of bullying, with 67% of teens who are online almost constantly reporting being a target of cyberbullying compared with 53% of those who use the internet less frequently.[3]

Although there is evidence that traditional and cyberbullying often occur together, there remains debate concerning how distinct these types of bullying are.[4] Taken together, at least moderate levels of bullying are estimated to occur in about 30% of school age children, although estimates vary widely because of differences in definition and methodology.[5] A recent study of 13 European and Asian countries found a nearly identical rate of overall victimization of 29.6%, although marked differences were found from one country to the next.[6] One piece of good news, however, is that there is evidence that the prevalence of bullying in the United States may be decreasing,[7] despite headlines to the contrary. A report from the Department of Education cites a rate of bullying at school of 22%, the lowest level since the data were gathered in 2005 (http://nces.ed.gov/blogs/nces/post/measuring-student-safety-bullying-rates-at-school).

School grounds remain the most common site for bullying (other than cyberbullying), and physical appearance is the most common target of bullying behavior.[8] Sexual orientation is also a common focus. Boys tend to bully more than girls, although this difference is diminished, if not reversed, when the definition includes more relational types of bullying.[9] Furthermore, boys tend to be more likely to bully those outside of their core group of friends, whereas girls are more likely to bully individuals within their social network.

Longitudinal studies reveal distinct patterns regarding bullying through childhood and adolescence. Early bullying can be readily identified in elementary school children but tends to peak in the middle school years and early adolescence. It often diminishes later in adolescence and adulthood, although there remains a minority of youth who increase their level of bullying through adolescence.[10]

Many studies of bullying have traditionally divided groups of children into those who are (1) bullies only, (2) victims only, and those who are (3) both bullies and victims. Other groups that are occasionally identified are bystanders, defenders, assistors, and reinforcers.[11] Although broad terms, such as bullies, are admittedly overly heterogeneous,[12] efforts have been slow to identify potentially more meaningful subtypes and categories. For example, there may be a group of more "alpha" bullies who tend to be popular, more socially dominant, and with less comorbid psychopathology in contrast to another group of bullies who are more dysregulated ("delta" bullies), less socially skilled, and with more associated behavioral and cognitive problems. Such distinctions could prove meaningful with regard to future research studies and intervention strategies.

NEGATIVE EFFECTS OF BULLYING

The negative effects of bullying are being increasingly appreciated. Indeed, bullying has been cited as one of the principle causes for the recent increase in depressive/anxiety symptoms and suicides that have been noted over the past decade among youth.[13] Although bullying as the root of our youth's declining mental health remains debated, the research is clear regarding its negative impact. Bullying is estimated to cause children to miss approximately 160,000 days of school each year according to the National Education Association (http://www.ncpc.org/topics/bullying/what-parents-can-do). A loss of up to 1.5 letter grades due to bullying has also been documented during the middle school years.[14] In the area of mental health and psychiatric disorders, bullying has been linked to future levels of anxiety, depression, suicidality, psychosis, and self-harm behaviors, among others.[15,16] And although the link has yet to be firmly established, bullying has been frequently invoked in the lead up to mass shooting events.[17] Overall, the level of trauma with regard to bullying has been found to be roughly equivalent to a child being placed outside of the home[18] and may be more severe than other forms of child maltreatment.[19] Outside of direct psychiatric illness, bullying in childhood has also been associated with higher levels of chronic inflammation in adulthood.[20]

The picture is more mixed with regard to the relations between bullies and mental health problems. Some studies have demonstrated that many bullies, especially those who also have been bully-victims, show elevated levels of psychopathology. Other studies, however, show evidence that more "pure" bullies may have relatively low rates of mental health problems.[21]

BULLYING DETECTION AND INTERVENTION

Many organizations including the American Academy of Pediatrics (AAP) and the American Academy of Child and Adolescent Psychiatry have emphasized the role of mental health professionals and other health care providers in reducing and preventing bullying. Giving anticipatory guidance, using effective tools to screen for bullying and making efforts in early intervention can lead to marked differences in the lives of many children and their families.

This section discusses methods to help identify bullies and their victims and then presents an overview of prevention strategies both at the individual and at the community level. One useful resource for clinicians is the Connected Kids Web site from the AAP (www.aap.org/), which provides information about screening, family guidance, and bullying interventions with a focus on violence prevention in routine health care visits.

Identification

A first step in preventing bullying is effective identification. Interventions against bullying start with early detection, as shown in **Box 1**. Often bullying is subtle and hidden, especially with regard to more covert relational bullying. It is also important to keep in mind that children often underreport bullying because of a fear of repercussions or feelings of disempowerment and shame.

When bullying victims do present for help, it is often in the context of general somatic complaints without an obvious cause. Victims may also show symptoms of

---

Box 1
Opportunities for bullying prevention in pediatric primary care (middle childhood)

1. Screen for bullying risk factors including sudden reports of changes in behavior (more depressed, suicidal ideation), truancy, and chronic somatic symptoms without a discernible cause.

2. Provide anticipatory guidance for elementary school students, especially those at risk (perceived as anxious, weaker than other children) before the peak bullying age in middle school. See section on individual level interventions for details.

3. Discuss openly, directly, and gently a child's experience at school. Do not dispute a child's report of bullying even if it is not perceived by parents or teachers.

4. Advocate for schools to adopt elements of effective bullying prevention programs.

---

social phobia, depression, or attention problems. They may also experience poorer grades or begin missing school.[22]

If bullying is suspected, further questions are warranted, which may include inquiries found in **Box 2**. Such questions can open the topic and reveal possible avenues for intervention, such as a more focused pediatric psychiatric referral or a discussion with the school principal to advocate for effective school-based interventions. For some children who seem reluctant to discuss their own personal history about bullying, initial questions that refer to the general climate of the school (eg, "Is bullying a problem at your school?") can sometimes help begin a conversation. It may also be worthwhile to remind young patients about the protection and limits of confidential discussions.

If more detailed information is needed, several screening and assessment tools are available. The Centers for Disease Control has published a compendium of instruments that are freely available to use to assess potential bullies, victims, and bully-victims.[23]

Individual-Level Interventions for Bully-Victims

Once bullying is suspected or uncovered, there are some general principles that can guide individual-level interventions in the office. Clinicians may find it helpful to

---

Box 2
Sample bullying screening questions

- I'd like to hear about how school is going. How many good friends do you have in school? (Child) Is your child being picked on at school? (Parent)

- Do you ever feel afraid to go to school? Why?

- Do other kids ever bully you at school, in your neighborhood or online? Who bullies you? When and where does it happen? What do they say or do?

- What do you do if you see other kids being bullied?

- Who can you go to for help if you or someone you know is being bullied?

- When you go for help, what is done about it?

Data from US Department of Health & Human Services. How to talk about bullying. Available at: www.stopbullying.gov. Accessed August 7, 2015.

---

differentiate lower levels of bullying (name calling, teasing) from higher levels (overt threats, physical violence, and intimidation), keeping in mind that all forms can be potentially harmful.

For lower level bullying, the following points are helpful to remember when working with kids directly and in helping parents help their children:

- Do not underestimate the power of sympathetic listening. Overt expressions to a child that he or she does not deserve this and that such behaviors are really hurtful can be very important to many kids. Positive experiences with friends and families can also go a long way to counteract a negative encounter with a bully.
- Coach bully-victims about how to respond. The old adage of telling a bully that he or she is hurting your feelings has been replaced with advice to react calmly and simply state one's disapproval of the bully's words or behavior or to leave the situation if possible. Some children also are helped by rehearsing specific responses or learning to join nonthreatening peer groups during higher risk activities.
- Engaging a child in general health promotion activities can be helpful. One study from the National Youth Risk Behavior Survey found that regular exercise (4 or more days a week) was associated with a 23% reduction in suicidal ideation among bullied students.[24]
- With cyberbullying, a discussion about Internet breaks or time away from social media platforms may seem a natural suggestion in order to limit a child's risk for exposure. There may, however, be some hazards to this approach, given the growing dependence on social media for educational and other communication needs and fears from adolescents of restriction. Rather than institute new limits, which may feel as a punishment and prevent disclosure of bullying behavior in the future, encouragement to save and report the offensive material may be preferable.
- Consider the option of an anonymous report to a school principal or guidance counselor. As an example, although school personnel may be unable to make a direct response, they might be able to provide more monitoring at high-risk areas, such as bathrooms, school buses, or locker rooms.

For higher levels of bullying, the role of the school, parents, and sometimes even law enforcement is more prominent. The government Web site www.stopbullying.gov/ includes several helpful suggestions and guidelines. Although the response in these instances may often be similar to lower level bullying, adults have a greater responsibility to determine what has happened and to design a response for the bully, if indicated. Many states now have mandatory bullying prevention and intervention policies. Although parents of bullying victims may have strong and natural urges to confront directly the parents of the alleged bully, this step often does not help the situation and can make things worse. Finally, if there is evidence that bullying is having a strong negative impact on the child, a more in-depth evaluation to rule out anxiety disorders, depression, posttraumatic stress disorder, and the presence of any suicidal or homicidal thinking is strongly considered.

Bullies

More evidence-based guidance is needed on how to identify and intervene with bullies individually. Keeping in mind that many youth who bully have histories of victimization and comorbid psychopathology, some may benefit from further evaluation and treatment. Alerting parents to bullying behavior and considering a referral for parent behavioral training can also be useful, although it should not be assumed that bullies necessarily come from dysfunctional households. According to some experts, common interventions that may exacerbate the harms associated with bullying include group therapy, "zero tolerance" approaches involving suspension or expulsion, or mediation sessions between the victim and bully.

Recently, the tide of intervention for bullies has focused on positive parenting. Positive parenting includes many elements associated with an authoritative parenting style that includes good communication, warmth, and respect, along with good levels of parental supervision. It also avoids harsher modes of discipline and criticism. Positive parenting has been found to have significant, albeit modest, preventative associations with bullying.[25] In addition, there is evidence that promoting increased empathy for the victim is more effective than condemning the bully's behaviors. In a randomized study of hundreds of children in 28 schools, it was found that bullies who were approached with a focus on building empathy for the victim rather than a strict condemnatory approach developed more insight and intention to stop their bullying behaviors.[26]

Taken together, there is evidence that some prevention of bullying is possible by parents and other adults through the cultivation of empathy.

School- and Community-Based Programs

Several comprehensive strategies for prevention and intervention of bullying behavior have been developed, including those that target cyberbullying and programs directed specifically toward bullies, victims, bystanders, teachers, educators, community members, families, and health care practitioners. In the context of bullying as a public health problem, many efforts are directed changing cultural attitudes, with strategies that target the social climate of schools and the greater community.

One of the pioneers in bullying research is Dan Olweus, a researcher on this topic since the 1970s at the University of Bergen in Norway. His work was inspired by several tragic adolescent deaths by suicide that were linked to bullying. The Olweus Bullying Prevention Program is arguably the most researched and widely adopted bullying prevention program in the world.[2] Its aim is to create a supportive school climate through repeated surveys of the school climate from staff, parents, and students. The program recommends the use of varied interventions that include group meetings and interactive videos to foster this change in climate over time.

The degree to which various antibullying programs have been scrutinized and tested varies considerably. The early literature on systematic bullying interventions tended to show improvement in knowledge and attitudes about bullying with little change in actual behavior.[27]

More recent meta-analyses of school-based antibullying programs have been more promising in finding that programs on average were effective at reducing bullying by around 20%.[28,29] Although research has not identified a specific program that has demonstrated superiority, universal programs seem to be as effective as more targeted interventions. Larger effect sizes have also been associated with more comprehensive multifaceted programs and those that reach out to students and use peer involvement.[30] Antibullying program can also be cost-effective, with a study done with the Finnish KiVa program estimating that their teacher administered program saved an estimated $66,172 over 50 years in their group of 200 students.[31]

CURRENT CONTROVERSIES AND SUMMARY

Although consensus continues to move forward regarding issues related to bullying and bullying intervention, there remain areas that are controversial and debated.

Even the definition of bullying is under scrutiny. The Global Health Initiative for the Prevention of Bullying (http://www.ghipb.org/definition-of-bullying.html), for example, disputes the requirement for intentionality and would include, under bullying, aggressive acts that are the results of a person being impulsive or dysregulated. The conceptualization of a bully is also under debate between the view of bullies as symptomatic individuals who themselves are suffering from mental health problems and the portrayal of bullies as more socially dominant individuals who use a *strategy* to maintain their rank within the peer community. Further research is needed to examine potentially meaningful subtypes when it comes to bullies and bully-victims.

With regard to intervention, there does seem to be some tension between the desire of schools and communities to demonstrate that they take bullying seriously while incorporating the increased recognition that purely punitive approaches to bullying are lacking in effectiveness. At the other end of the spectrum, interventions that involve the bully and victim directly meeting to work out their problems with the help of an adult or even peer mediator are no less controversial, with some experts finding this intervention both ineffective and potentially traumatic for the victim, similar to situations of domestic violence.[32]

It is clear from the research that there is no quick and easy solution to bullying. Clinicians of all types can reduce trauma and help patients and families on the individual level while advocating for effective programs for the broader community. Research suggests that many of the most successful programs incorporate all students in a school universally and promote long-term shifts in the school culture that can only occur with broad participation from students, staff, parents, community members, and families. Nevertheless, there remains much to learn on many levels about bullying and the ways that this important public health issue can be more fully addressed and prevented.

FINANCIAL DISCLOSURE

Dr D.C. Rettew reports royalties from Oxford University Press and Psychology Today and is a consultant to Happy Health, Inc. Dr S. Pawlowski reports no financial relationships with commercial interests.

REFERENCES

1. Rettew DC, Pawlowski S. Bullying. Child Adolesc Psychiatry Clin N Am 2016; 25(2):235–42.
2. Olweus D. Bullying at school: what it is and what we can do. Cambridge (United Kingdom): Blackwell; 1993.
3. Anderson M. A majority of teens have experienced some form of cyberbulling. Pew Research Center. 2018. Available at: https://www.pewresearch.org/internet/2018/09/27/a-majority-of-teens-have-experienced-some-form-of-cyberbullying/. Accessed June 28, 2021.
4. Tzani-Pepelasi C, Ioannou M, Synnott J, et al. Comparing factors related to school-bullying and cyber-bullying. Crime Psychol Rev 2018;4(1):1–25.
5. Nansel TR, Overpeck M, Pilla RS, et al. Bullying behaviors among US youth: prevalence and association with psychosocial adjustment. JAMA 2001;285(16): 2094–100.
6. Chudal R, Tiiri E, Brunstein Klomek A, et al. Victimization by traditional bullying and cyberbullying and the combination of these among adolescents in 13 European and Asian countries. Eur Child Adolesc Psychiatry 2021. https://doi.org/10.1007/s00787-021-01779-6.

7. Finkelhor D, Turner HA, Shattuck A, et al. Prevalence of childhood exposure to violence, crime, and abuse: results from the national survey of children's exposure to violence. JAMA Pediatr 2015;169(8):746–54.

8. Davis S, Nixon CL. Youth voice project: student insights into bullying and peer mistreatment. Champaign (IL): Research Press Publishers; 2015.

9. Coyne SM, Archer J, Elsea M. "We're not friends anymore unless.": the frequency and harmfulness of indirect, relational, and social aggression. Aggress Behav 2006;32:294–307.

10. Pepler D, Jiang D, Craig W, et al. Developmental trajectories of bullying and associated factors. Child Dev 2008;79(2):325–38.

11. Huitsing G, Veenstra R. Bullying in classrooms: participant roles from a social network perspective. Aggress Behav 2012;38(6):494–509.

12. Vaillancourt T, Hymel S, McDougall P. Bullying is power: implications for school-based intervention strategies. J Appl Sch Psychol 2003;19:157–76.

13. Twenge JM, Cooper AB, Joiner TE, et al. Age, period, and cohort trends in mood disorder indicators and suicide-related outcomes in a nationally representative dataset, 2005-2017. J Abnorm Psychol 2017;128(3):185–99.

14. Juvonen J, Wang Y, Espinoza G. Bullying experiences and compromised academic performance across middle school grades. J Early Adolesc 2011;31(1):152–73.

15. Arseneault L, Walsh E, Trzesniewski K, et al. Bullying victimization uniquely contributes to adjustment problems in young children: a nationally representative cohort study. Pediatrics 2006;118(1):130–8.

16. Wolke D, Copeland WE, Angold A, et al. Impact of bullying in childhood on adult health, wealth, crime, and social outcomes. Psychol Sci 2013;24(10):1958–70.

17. Leary MR, Kowalski RM, Smith L, et al. Teasing, rejection, and violence: case studies in the school shootings. Aggressive Behav 2003;29:202–14.

18. Takizawa R, Maughan B, Arseneault L. Adult health outcomes of childhood bullying victimization: evidence from a five-decade longitudinal British birth cohort. Am J Psychiatry 2014;171(7):777–84.

19. Copeland WE, Wolke D, Angold A, et al. Adult psychiatric outcomes of bullying and being bullied by peers in childhood and adolescence. JAMA Psychiatry 2013;70(4):419–26.

20. Copeland WE, Wolke D, Lereya ST, et al. Childhood bullying involvement predicts low-grade systemic inflammation into adulthood. Proc Natl Acad Sci U S A 2014; 111(21):7570–5.

21. Koh JB, Wong JS. Survival of the fittest and the sexiest: evolutionary origins of adolescent bullying. J Interpers Violence 2015;32(17):2668–90.

22. Zimmerman FJ, Glew GM, Christakis DA, et al. Early cognitive stimulation, emotional support, and television watching as predictors of subsequent bullying among grade-school children. Arch Pediatr Adolesc Med 2005;159(4):384–8.

23. Hamburger ME, Basile KC, Vivolo AM. Measuring bullying victimization, perpetration, and bystander experiences: a compendium of assessment tools. Atlanta, GA: Centers for Disease Control and Prevention, National Center for Injury Prevention and Control; 2011.

24. Sibold J, Edwards E, Murray-Close D, et al. Physical activity, sadness, and suicidality in bullied US adolescents. J Am Acad Child Adolesc Psychiatry 2015; 54(10):808–15.

25. Leyera ST, Samara M, Wolke D. Parenting behavior and the risk of becoming a victim and a bully/victim: a meta analysis study. Child Abuse Negl 2013;37(12): 1091–108.

26. Garandeau CF, Vartio A, Poskiparta E, et al. School bullies' intention to change behavior following teacher interventions: effects of empathy arousal, condemning of bullying, and blaming of the perpetrator. Prev Sci 2016;17(8):1034–43.
27. Merrell KW, Gueldner BA, Ross SW, et al. How effective are school bullying intervention programs? A meta-analysis of intervention research. Sch Psychol Q 2008; 23(1):26–42.
28. Gaffney H, Ttofi MM, Farrington DP. Evaluating the effectiveness of school bullying prevention programs: an updated meta-analytic review. Agg Viol Behav 2019;45:111–33.
29. Fraguas D, Díaz-Caneja CM, Ayora M, et al. Assessment of school anti-bullying interventions: a meta-analysis of randomized controlled trials. JAMA Pediatr 2021;175(1):44–55.
30. Gaffney H, Ttofi MM, Farrington DP. What works in anti-bullying programs? Analysis of effective intervention components. J Sch Psychol 2021;85:37–56.
31. McDaid D, Park AL, Wahlbeck K. The economic case for the prevention of mental illness. Annu Rev Public Health 2019;40:373–89.
32. Cohen R. Stop mediating these conflicts now! The school mediator: peer mediation insights from the desk of Richard Cohen. Watertown, MA: School Mediation Associates Electronic Newsletter; 2002. Available at: www.schoolmediation.com. Accessed August 7, 2015.

Social Media as It Interfaces with Psychosocial Development and Mental Illness in Transitional-Age Youth

Brian A. Primack, MD, PhD[a],*, Kristi L. Perryman, PhD[a],
Rachael A. Crofford, MS[a], César G. Escobar-Viera, MD, PhD[b]

KEYWORDS

- Social media • Depression • Anxiety • Facebook • Emotional contagion
- Cognitive neuroscience • Sleep • Social networks

KEY POINTS

- Social media has grown substantially, with more than 4.2 billion new users worldwide in the past 25 years.
- Nearly all transitional-age youth use social media, and most use it daily.
- Social media use has increased during the time of COVID-19.
- Large nationally representative studies demonstrate consistent, linear associations between social media use and depression and anxiety among young adults.
- However, social media networks also may be leveraged to identify individuals with mental health concerns and engage transitional-age youth in treatment.
- Future research will be important to determine best practices for optimal use of social media to retain its benefits but minimize its drawbacks.

INTRODUCTION
Definition and Scope of Social Media

Social media (SM) can be defined as "a group of Internet-based applications that allow the creation and exchange of user-generated content."[1] This includes formation of online communities and sharing of information, ideas, opinions, messages, images, and videos. Therefore, although all online video games would not necessarily count as SM, video games that allow for substantial sharing of information and development of online communities do fit this definition. SM has become an integral component of how people worldwide connect with friends and family, share personal content, and obtain

[a] College of Education and Health Professions, University of Arkansas, Fayetteville, AR 72701, USA; [b] Department of Psychiatry, University of Pittsburgh School of Medicine, Pittsburgh, PA 15213, USA
* Corresponding author.
E-mail address: bprimack@uark.edu

Child Adolesc Psychiatric Clin N Am 31 (2022) 11–30
https://doi.org/10.1016/j.chc.2021.07.007
1056-4993/22/© 2021 Elsevier Inc. All rights reserved.

news and entertainment.[2,3] Use of SM is particularly prevalent among transitional-age youth (TAY), usually defined as individuals aged 16 to 24 years, who are at critical junctures around developmental tasks such as identity development and establishment of social norms.[4]

Currently, the most commonly used SM platform is Facebook[3,5,6]; however, there are many other commonly used SM sites, such as YouTube, Twitter, TikTok, Instagram, WhatsApp, SnapChat, Pinterest, and Reddit.[7] Furthermore, various SM platforms lend themselves to different types of communication and applications.[8] For example, many TAY maintain Facebook accounts but use them primarily for posting photos and receiving information from formal groups, such as college-related activities. These individuals may use Instagram or SnapChat instead for private conversations with close friends. Meanwhile, Twitter and Reddit are common sources of news, whereas LinkedIn can be important for occupational social networking. Finally, sites such as Pinterest tend to be more popular among individuals with cooking, artistic, and/or craft-related aspirations.

Growth of Social Media

It is difficult to overstate the rapid growth of SM use. Many people consider the birth of modern SM to be in the mid- to late-1990s, with a platform called SixDegrees. The subsequent decade was marked by the success of MySpace and the emergence of multiple other platforms. However, it was not until the mid-2000s that today's most frequently used sites, such as Facebook and Twitter, became more mainstream. In 2020, it was estimated that 4.2 billion individuals used SM worldwide.[9] This represents a greater-than-90% increase in SM use globally since 2015.

Use has been particularly high among TAY. For example, in the United States, approximately 84% of young adults aged 18 to 29 years use SM, and most users visit these sites at least once a day.[2,3] About 95% of youth aged 13 to 17 years own smartphones, and nearly all of them use SM.[2,3] However, use in other age groups is also substantially increasing. For example, use among adults aged 65 years and older in the United States grew from 34% to 45% between 2016 and 2021.[9] Overall, average SM use by Internet users worldwide is estimated at 145 minutes per day.[2,3]

Globally, Facebook currently maintains approximately 2.7 billion users,[2] which makes its population approximately 8 times that of the United States. The next most widely used SM platform is YouTube with 2.3 billion users.[2] WhatsApp has 2 billion users, Facebook Messenger has 1.3 billion users, Instagram has 1.2 billion users, and WeChat has 1.2 million users.[2] It is important to note that platform usage differs significantly by age. For example, adults aged 30 years and older tend to use Facebook and YouTube, whereas TAY more commonly use Instagram, SnapChat, and TikTok.[3]

Coronavirus Pandemic

In December 2019, the United States, along with the rest of the world, began to experience the effects of the outbreak of the coronavirus pandemic (COVID-19). This included substantial morbidity and mortality and the shutdown of schools, places of worship, restaurants, and other public facilities. Many families transitioned to work and education at home. The resulting social isolation, along with the necessity of more time on the computer to complete school, likely resulted in more time on SM for TAY.[10]

Preliminary research indicates that mental health problems increased substantially among adolescents during the pandemic. For example, a study conducted in China found that, during the COVID-19 outbreak, individuals aged 12 to 18 years had a

43% likelihood of depression, 37% anxiety, and 31% with both, and these numbers are much higher than usual.[11]

However, the net influence of SM during the pandemic is unclear. On the one side, SM usually is associated with psychological distress, depression, and anxiety.[12] However, SM may also have facilitated positive social and school connections. Time out of school is associated with increased screen time, irregular sleep patterns, decreased physical activity, and a less healthy diet, all of which increase adolescents' risk for mental health issues.[13] While well-controlled long-term research on the impact of the pandemic on SM use is still underway, this review will include studies published to the current time related to COVID-19.

Social Media, Mental Illness, and the Purpose of This Review

Any rapid social and behavioral change is likely to influence mental health. There has been a fair amount of research exploring how SM interfaces with both psychosocial development and mental health conditions among young adults. We aim in this article to broadly summarize major understandings that have been gleaned to date and to summarize important future directions for research. Because of the continuously emerging situation related to COVID-19, which for reasons described earlier may relate to both SM use and emotional health conditions among transition-age individuals, we carefully assessed literature published by May 1, 2021, the last feasible date to complete this review.

PUBLISHED LITERATURE AROUND SOCIAL MEDIA, DEVELOPMENT, AND MENTAL HEALTH
Neuroscience and Developmental Psychology Around Social Media

The rapid growth of SM, as well as several studies showing an increasing time spent on SM sites among adolescents and young adults, has generated interest In the potential impact of SM on the developing brain of adolescents and young adults.[6,8,12–14] However, few rigorous studies have focused on this area to date. A recently published review found only 11 articles covering the topic with adolescents aged 11 to 18 years between 2012 and 2020.[15] One study used functional MRI to analyze social cognition and social influences.[16] Researchers measured activity in neural regions of adolescents, while they were looking at a simulated Instagram like feed of images. The findings showed that adolescents were more inclined to "like" photos that already had been "liked" many times. Additionally, there was a positive association between the number of "likes" seen and activity of neural regions usually linked to attention, imitation, social cognition, and reward processing.[16] According to the investigators, these findings suggest that SM may trigger a unique type of peer pressure through quantifiable social endorsement, which in turn might reinforce the importance of self-presentation during adolescence, including on SM.[16]

There are also observations from related work that may be relevant.[17] For example, because of its mobility and tendency to provide interruptions, SM use may be associated with increased multitasking, which has been linked with negative cognitive and mental health outcomes.[18,19] For example, multitasking has been related to decreased ability to sustain attention,[20,21] poor academic performance,[22–24] decreased subjective well-being,[25] and higher levels of depression and anxiety.[26,27] It will be valuable for future research to examine more closely associations between SM use and pathways to these outcomes via multitasking.

SM messages tend to be brief and to link to multiple other sources. This may affect the ability to pay attention, which has also been associated with negative mental health outcomes. Because individuals in the United States use SM for approximately 2 to 3 hours per day,[28] this may present a substantial challenge, especially for youth who already have attention problems.

Other research has linked increased use of technology and Internet to aggression and desensitization to pain and suffering. For example, one study used functional MRI to evaluate the impact of Internet use and video games in older adolescents.[29] Because their findings showed suppressed activation of the amygdala during portrayal of violent imagery, the investigators surmise that exposure to these messages may be associated with an increase in aggressive behavior during adulthood.[29] It is not clear whether these speculations extend to SM as well.

On the other hand, some studies have suggested benefits of SM use for some adolescents, especially those lacking in social skills.[30] Prolonged SM use may positively affect adolescent affective and cognitive empathy, broadening the ability to express the feelings and appreciate feelings of others. Video games have also been associated with certain improvements in visual, cognitive, attention, and motor skills.[31] For example, avid video game players may exhibit better visual memory and were flexible in switching between tasks.[31] Therefore, it will be valuable for future work to determine if these related findings extend to SM in terms of its potential for affecting both positive and negative developmental and cognitive outcomes.

Benefits and Concerns Around Social Media to Provide Mental Health Treatment

SM may present opportunities to augment traditional mental health treatment. For example, researchers have used publicly available SM data to provide surveillance and determine if patients are exhibiting suicidal and/or psychotic behavior.[32–35] However, this type of surveillance has also been criticized as a potential invasion of patients' privacy.[32,34]

SM and related Internet tools—such as telepsychiatry and mobile apps—may also provide useful alternatives to traditional clinical care. This is particularly the case because factors such as stigma, logistics, and finances have been identified as important barriers to mental health care. Thus, especially for those of transitional age who are highly accustomed to using SM, accessing care in this way may help lift those barriers.

The outbreak of COVID-19 in 2019—and all the mental health issues that surfaced because of the associated fear, anxiety, and social isolation—resulted in a rapid transition for mental health professionals to virtual or remote care. The Centers for Medicare & Medicaid Services (CMS) and the Substance Abuse and Mental Health Services Administration (SAMHSA) established practice guidance that included information on the impact of the pandemic on minoritized groups, telepsychiatry, and billing.[36] These guidelines were adopted by the American Psychiatric Association (APA) as part of their COVID-19 practice guidance.[37] Some prior requirements related to HIPAA, prior authorization, and referral were waived to quickly transition to virtual mental health services. Research on the impact of telepsychiatry services during the pandemic is limited. A recent systematic review used a PubMed search for peer-reviewed research from January 1990 to March 2020.[38] Themes that emerged from this study included privacy and legal issues, advantages and disadvantages of telepsychiatry, treatment of psychiatric disorders and psychotherapy via telepsychiatry, and modern technologies in mental health care.[38] Advantages included improved access to care, safety and comfort using devices, ability to receive services in native languages without an interpreter, and improved access to services.[38]

Concerns about the provision of mental health care using SM and telepsychiatry services existed before the pandemic. For example, therapeutic relationships formed over SM networks may be inferior to those developed using person-to-person interactions.[39] Second, therapists are trained to use many nonverbal cues and language in their assessments. Other important issues are related to professional liability ramifications tied to the provision of treatment over SM. Finally, it will ultimately be important and practical for mental health professionals to understand reimbursement models and billing requirements for these services.

Other concerns that have emerged since COVID-19 include inability of the mental health professionals to take physical action to help their patients, interruptions caused by technical difficulties, and the lack of mental health professionals trained specifically for telepsychiatric services.[38]

Benefits and Concerns Around Social Media to Provide Social Support and Education Among Individuals with Mental Illness

SM may facilitate forming connections among people with potentially stigmatizing health disorders, including depression, anxiety, schizophrenia, and autism spectrum disorders (ASDs).[40–44] This may happen over traditional SM sites, such as Facebook, Reddit, and Tumblr. However, there are also specialized SM sites related to mental health, such as "Together All" (www.togetherall.com) and "Mental Health is Health" (www.mentalhealthis-health.us). These sites, which offer the ability for individuals with mental health concerns to support each other, emphasize factors such as respecting privacy and confidentiality.[45] There are also Web sites from organizations such as the National Alliance on Mental Illness that educate about mental illness and provide a helpline conferring information and support for those struggling with mental health issues, including peer-to-peer support services.[46]

SM can also facilitate self-disclosures that can provide education, support, and comfort to individuals with mental health concerns.[47] TAY who are comfortable with SM platforms find these interventions engaging, accessible, and value the support they provide.[48] The average user will often not self-disclose potentially stigmatizing information such as struggling with a mental illness.[49] However, a growing number of individuals post self-disclosures around mental illness.[49–51] The information these individuals post may provide high-quality resources around mental health and spark valuable conversations.[49–51]

A study conducted with 25 transitional-age participants on Tumblr who had posted about depression demonstrated that receiving online mental health resources was associated with greater satisfaction.[52] A different study focused on 165 Instagram, Twitter, Facebook, Reddit, Tumblr, and online depression forum participants who had major depression and had symptoms in the past 2 weeks about depression-related topics. They found that online platforms were an effective way to recruit participants who want mental health support.[47]

Mental health messages can come from ordinary users or from "virtual celebrities," who make their livelihood by posting material online. Because these videos can have millions of views, when the information provided in these videos is accurate, they can be valuable to the public for three reasons. First, they may provide information to individuals who do not have access to health care professionals,[47] either for logistical reasons or due to embarrassment. Second, peer-to-peer education and support are known to improve mental and physical well-being.[48] Third, these messages can demystify these previously stigmatizing conditions.[48]

However, there remain concerns if the information provided is not accurate.[39] A high-profile example of this is the damage that was done by a prominent celebrity who prominently disseminated unsubstantiated concerns regarding vaccines and autism.[49] Additionally, self-disclosures during acute crises of mental disorders may lead to "oversharing," with potential consequences such as increased stigmatization and cyberbullying.[50–52] Moreover, use of temporary SM accounts, which provide some degree of anonymity, can be associated with problematic outcomes, such as higher negativity, cognitive bias, self-attention–seeking posts, and decreased self-esteem.[50–52] Semianonymity may thus fulfill a unique need, allowing users to express views and thoughts about a topic, such as depression, that is usually considered highly sensitive. There is also the potential for individuals to use SM to form bonds with each other around emotional concerns. It is an important developmental task of youth and young adults to form peer relationships, and SM may facilitate this. However, there also are questions as to whether online social contact with family members or close friends is a more productive way to approach the development of social relationships than with strangers and acquaintances.[53,54] A recent study looked to address this question and found that face-to-face emotional support was associated with lower odds of depression than social media–based support.[55] This finding was further corroborated in a study that examined the real-life relationship individuals had with their SM contacts. It found that having no face-to-face relationship with social media contacts was associated with increased symptoms of depression, while close relationships with SM contacts was associated with decreased symptoms of depression.[56]

Population-Level Monitoring of Mental Health Concerns

Researchers have capitalized on readily available SM data to learn about human behavior and social phenomena. For example, SM data show promise for prediction of political election results.[57,58] SM data also have been useful in monitoring health-related issues, such as disaster response to earthquakes[59] and outbreaks such as influenza.[60–62] Therefore, there has been interest in leveraging these tools to better understand mental health. For example, some researchers have used SM data to better understand factors surrounding suicide attempts.[63,64] A recent systematic review identified current evidence on utilization of SM as a tool for suicide prevention. After analyzing 30 studies, the investigators found most studies were descriptive or qualitative and that no studies had reported on actual interventions. These findings underscore the need for more empirical research. They also suggest that SM platforms can be accessed by a large number of otherwise-difficult-to-engage participants, providing an anonymous, yet accessible and nonjudgmental environment. Ultimately, this may allow interventions to be conducted after an expression of suicidal ideation is made online.[65]

Data from focus groups conducted among SM users with and without depression suggest that there is a wide range of reactions to this type of research. Although many individuals appreciate the value of using public domain information as a resource to improve mental health monitoring, others are concerned about issues related to privacy and lack of oversight.[66]

A systematic review assessed the validity of using social media markers for depression screening. The review included studies involving Facebook, Twitter, Instagram, and Snapchat profiles. While the reviewed studies used different methods, which made some comparisons challenging, the authors of the review were able to find criteria that indicated that screening social media profiles could be a valid way to detect depression.[67] Another study found that depressive symptoms change the way individuals use social media and may be helpful to identify the markers of someone who is at risk for depressive symptoms.[68]

Another study analyzed a random sample of 2000 tweets to assess depression-related content. Researchers found that although 40% of the chatter consisted of supportive or helpful tweets, 32% disclosed feelings of depression. More than 65% of all tweets contained one or more DSM-5 symptoms necessary for the diagnosis of a major depressive disorder. These findings underline the potential avenue that SM offers for prevention and awareness campaigns.[64]

Emotional Contagion

In-person interaction can be a powerful purveyor for "emotional contagion," resulting in the potential exacerbation and/or amelioration of emotional states. It is an important task of adolescence and young adulthood to develop identity based on shared interests and experiences.

There has been interest in determining whether this contagion effect applies in the SM milieu. One large study suggested that emotional states can be transferred among participants of SM via observation of others' positive experiences.[69] The investigators conducted an experiment among real Facebook users without their knowledge. They altered the amount of emotional material that was presented in certain users' News Feed and observed whether there were changes in participants' person-to-person interactions. They found that when positively valanced expressions were reduced, participants spontaneously produced fewer positive posts and more negative posts. They also found that when negative expressions were reduced, there were fewer negative posts and more positive posts. The investigators concluded that in-person interaction and nonverbal cues are not strictly necessary for emotional contagion.[69]

Research also suggests that the likelihood of feeling happy after reading a positive post on Facebook is significantly related to strength of the relationship between the 2 individuals.[70] Although this may seem intuitive, these findings are important because they suggest potential avenues for intervention. For example, if individuals can be encouraged to increase positive posts through intervention, this may decrease overall negative cognitions.

Social Media and Mental Health Outcomes Among Young Adults

There is controversy as to whether, among young adults, overall SM use is associated with mental health outcomes. Some studies suggest that SM users may experience an increase in social capital, perceived social support, and life satisfaction.[71,72] Similarly, use of SM may provide opportunities for keeping in touch with family and friends, as well as other social interactions that may increase social capital and alleviate mental health concerns, such as depression and anxiety.[71,73,74] However, large-scale cross-sectional epidemiologic studies conducted among this population tend to find associations between increased SM use and negative outcomes related to mental health, such as depression, anxiety, poor sleep, eating concerns, and poor emotional support.

Depression

Initial work examining associations between SM use and depression was cross-sectional. A nationally representative study based in the United States looked at individuals aged 19 to 32 years. It found consistent, linear associations between quartile of SM use and degree of depression as measured with the Patient-Reported Outcomes Measurement Information System (PROMIS) brief depression scale.[75] Results were consistent whether SM use was approximated by self-reported time spent on SM or by a frequency of use measure based on the Pew Internet Research study. For example, compared with those in the lowest quartile, individuals in the highest quartile of SM site visits per week had significantly increased odds of depression [adjusted odds ratio (AOR): 2.74, 95% confidence interval (CI): 1.86 to 4.04].[75] Similar findings have been reported internationally. For example, a study of 340 Lebanese medical students suggested that there was a significant association between depression and Facebook use, including the specific use of Facebook-related tools, such as the "like" and "add friend" buttons.[76] Additionally, a study of 467 Scottish adolescents, which examined SM use and its association with sleep, anxiety, and depression, found that those who used more SM had lower sleep quality, worse self-esteem, increased anxiety, and increased depression.[77]

Because these studies are cross-sectional, they do not help determine causality. For example, it may be that individuals who are depressed turn to SM to self-soothe. On the other hand, depressive cognitions may be triggered in frequent SM users. For example, frequent SM users may substitute SM for potentially more valuable face-to-face social interactions.[78,79] Alternatively, frequent exposure to highly curated, unrealistic portrayals on SM may give people the impression that others are living happier, more connected lives, which may make people feel more depressed in comparison.

More recent research confirms prior cross-sectional findings in the longitudinal setting. For example, a study published in 2020 explored temporal associations between depression and SM use.[80] In this study, SM use at baseline was strongly associated with the development of depression among nondepressed individuals over the subsequent 6 months. In fact, even while controlling for covariates, those in the highest quartile of SM use had about three times the odds for developing depression compared with those in the lowest quartile of SM use. However, interestingly, the presence of depression at baseline was not associated with an increase in SM use over the subsequent 6 months.[80] While no study can demonstrate causality, this temporal association between initial social media use and development of depression—without any indication of depression leading to increase SM use—was noteworthy.

Studies also suggest value in studying nuanced contextual factors of SM as they relate to depression. For example, one study found that negative experiences online were associated with *increased* depressive symptoms, whereas positive experiences were not associated with *decreased* depressive symptoms.[81] These results were consistent with "negativity bias," for which negative experiences can be more powerful than positive experiences. Another study found an association between social media dependence and depressive symptoms. The depressive symptoms were significant in university students that preferred Twitter instead of Instagram and Facebook.[82]

In a systematic review that explored whether youth use SM to share ideas and thoughts about deliberate self-harm, depressive language was present in 19% of participants.[65] This review also found a number of beneficial suggestions that were shared among SM users, such as ideas for formal treatment and advice on how to stop self-harming behavior. However, some concerning ideas were also shared, such as normalization of self-harming behavior, concealment of suicidal plans or ideas, and live enactments of self-harm acts.[83]

The positive and negative effects of SM are evident in specific populations as well. In the lesbian, gay, and bisexual (LGB) population, a systematic review found that SM can have both positive and negative effects when it comes to depression. The benefits of SM for LGB individuals can be decreased isolation and loneliness, while the negative effects can be increased cyberbullying and other SM usage patterns that are associated with depression.[84]

A meta-analysis examined the multidimensional constructs of SM use by reviewing depressive symptoms separately.[85] Symptoms included intensity of SM use, problematic SM use, and time spent using SM. The association between symptoms of depression to problematic SM use was moderate and was significantly higher than time spent using SM or intensity of SM use.[85] Symptoms of depression were significantly, though mildly, associated with time spent and intensity. Gender, age, year of study publication, and mode of recruitment were not significant moderates. Thus, more in-depth research focusing on individuals who are participating in problematic SM use would be beneficial.

Anxiety

A population-based study of Scottish adolescents also found associations between increased SM use and anxiety.[77] Also, an online survey conducted in Norway among 23,533 individuals aged 16 years and older found a positive and significant association between symptoms of anxiety and obsessive compulsive disorder and potentially addictive use of SM.[86] Another study based in the United States involved a sample of 243 college students. These researchers found that there were significant associations between problematic use of Facebook, social anxiety, and the need for social assurance.[87]

Poor sleep

Researchers examined a nationally representative sample of young adults and found that increased SM use was independently associated with poor sleep.[88] Sleep disturbance was assessed using the brief PROMIS sleep disturbance measure. In models that adjusted for all sociodemographic covariates, participants with higher SM use volume and frequency had significantly greater odds of having sleep disturbance. For example, compared with those in the lowest quartile of SM use per day, those in the highest quartile had an AOR of 1.95 (95% CI: 1.37–2.79) for sleep disturbance. Similarly, compared with those in the lowest quartile of SM use frequency per week, those in the highest quartile had an AOR of 2.92 (95% CI: 1.97–4.32) for sleep disturbance. All associations demonstrated a significant linear trend.[88]

Research has found consistent results among 467 Scottish adolescents; again increased SM use was associated with poor sleep.[77] In this study, the researchers also found that nighttime-specific SM use was associated with poorer sleep, even when models controlled for related mental health factors, such as anxiety, depression, and self-esteem.[77]

A recent study evaluated the impact of SM on the sleep of teenagers and the effects of sleep deprivation.[89] Researchers found that having access to SM is associated with reduced sleep, especially if teenagers have a cell phone in their room. They also found that this negatively impacted their mood and daily function and that this worsens as they age.

Eating concerns

Multiple concerns have been raised in the literature regarding the availability on SM sites of problematic content that encourages disordered eating behaviors. For example, there are many so-called "pro-anorexia" communities on SM that encourage eating behaviors that physical health professionals would consider extremely problematic and dangerous, such as severe calorie restriction.[90] However, it also has been noted in the literature that there is also a growing community of individuals on SM who post "anti–pro-anorexia" messages.[91] Therefore, it is valuable for clinicians who work with individuals who have eating disorders to understand the complex dynamic environment of SM around this particular issue. It has also been noted that pro-anorexia SM content can be influential with regard to male body image issues.[92]

One large, nationally representative study examined this issue on a population level instead of focusing on those under specific eating disorder criteria.[93] In particular, the researchers examined overall SM use and the likelihood of having more eating-related and body image–related concerns in general. They found that, compared with those in the lowest quartile, participants in the highest quartiles for SM use volume and frequency had significantly greater odds of having eating concerns (AOR: 2.18, 95% CI: 1.50–3.17 and AOR: 2.55, 95% CI: 1.72–3.78, respectively). There were significant positive overall linear associations between the SM use variables and eating concerns (P<.001).[93] Although this was a cross-sectional study and directionality could not be established, these findings suggest that unhealthy messages around body image and eating behaviors may be a concern even in general SM environments and not only in the more extreme cases.

Autism spectrum disorders
The literature regarding ASDs and SM is still emerging. Most studies are descriptive in nature.[94–96] Additionally, data have primarily been obtained from parents or caregivers, and most of these studies have focused solely on reporting prevalence of SM among people living with ASDs.[94–96] In general, these studies have found that although young adults with ASDs spend most of their free time using television or video games, only a small fraction uses SM in general.[94–96]

Emotional support
Some relatively small and localized studies indicate that frequent use of SM may be associated with declines in subjective well-being, life satisfaction, and real-life community.[97] These data are borne out in larger studies as well. For example, a nationally representative study of US young adults found that increased daily time devoted to SM use was independently associated with lower perceived emotional support. In particular, the researchers' multivariable model including all sociodemographic covariates and accounting for survey weights demonstrated that, compared with the lowest quartile of time on SM, being in the highest quartile was significantly associated with decreased odds of having higher perceived emotional support (AOR: 0.62, 95% CI: 0.40–0.94). Interestingly, however, this same study did not find a significant association with emotional support when SM was operationalized in terms of the number of sites visited per week.[28]

FUTURE DIRECTIONS
Need for Longitudinal Research
Although one strong longitudinal study has been published,[80] most data linking SM use and mental health outcomes have been cross-sectional. When a study finds that there is a broad association between SM use and depression, for example, this may indicate that individuals with depression tend to use more SM; depressed individuals with a diminished sense of self-worth may turn to SM-based interactions for validation.[98,99] Subsequently, individuals may suffer from continuous rumination and guilt surrounding Internet use, while feeling compelled to continue the cycle owing to low self-efficacy and negative self-appraisal.[98,100] Owing to the high accessibility of SM and the possibility of socialization in a controlled setting, individuals with underlying depression and anhedonia may be more drawn to SM interactions rather than to face-to-face interactions.[101,102] However, it also may be that those who use increased amounts of SM subsequently develop or increase depressive symptoms.

Multiple studies have linked SM use with declines in subjective mood, sense of well-being, and life satisfaction.[28,97,103] For example, passive consumption of SM content, as opposed to active communication, has been associated with decrease in bonding and bridging social capital and increase in loneliness.[103] One explanation may be that exposure to highly idealized representations of peers on SM elicits feelings of envy and the distorted belief that others lead happier and/or more successful lives. Consequently, these envious feelings may lead to a sense of self-inferiority and depression over time.[103] It is also possible that the feeling of "time wasted" by engaging in activities of little meaning on SM negatively influences mood.[103] Moreover, in a nationally representative survey that assessed general health among college-age students, Internet use and computer games have consistently been identified among the top 5 factors impacting their academic performance.[104] Additionally, the substantial increase in the amount of time young individuals spend on the Internet, particularly on SM, has led some to call for the recognition of "Internet addiction" as a distinct psychiatric condition that is closely associated with depression.[105,106] This consideration is more crucial with the influence of the pandemic on SM use. Finally, it is possible that increased SM exposure may increase the risk of cyberbullying, which also may increase symptoms of depression.[107]

Need for Clinically Based Research

Because most research in this area has focused on community-based populations, it will be valuable for future work to involve clinical populations to facilitate discoveries with clinically relevant conclusions. For example, discovery of associations between SM use and mental disorders suggests that it may be valuable for clinicians to assess SM use among depressed individuals to probe for maladaptive patterns of use, which may be contributing to mood dysregulation. However, clinicians are extremely busy, and the actual value of this additional task has not been systematically studied. Still, because SM use is so common and integral to TAY, bringing up a discussion of SM use would seem to have potential value simply in getting to know a patient better.

Because SM has become an integral component of human interaction, it is important for clinicians interacting with young adults to recognize the important balance to be struck in encouraging potential positive use but redirecting from problematic use. Although much of the high-profile research has found overall associations between SM use and mental health problems, suggesting major limitation of use may be viewed by patients as insensitive or misguided.

Use of Social Media to Screen for Mental Health Problems

There may be useful ways of leveraging SM to identify individuals at risk, such as detecting self-disclosures of depression on SM.[51,52] The teams behind some SM sites have already begun to reach out to users who show signs of mental disorders. At one point, when one searched blog site Tumblr for tags indicative of a mental health crisis, such as "depressed," "suicidal," or "hopeless," the search function redirected to a message that began with "Everything okay?" and provided links to pertinent resources. Similarly, Facebook has tested a feature by which users' friends could anonymously report worrisome posts. Authors of problematic content received pop-up messages on their next visit to the site voicing concern and encouraging them to speak with a friend or helpline worker.

Continued research into the factors that relate SM and depression will allow sites to refine these procedures and reach out to those with greatest potential need. This is especially critical given the increased risk of suicide since the COVID-19 pandemic. A recent study examined suicide risk among 11- to 21-year-olds from January to July 2020.[108] Suicidal ideation was significantly higher in March and July of 2020, with higher rates of attempts of suicide in February, March, April, and July 2020 than in the same months in the previous year. The mean age of participants in the study was 14.72 years, with 47.7% Latinx, 26.7% white, and 18.7% Black.[108] This is likely an indicator of the stress and social isolation felt by TAY during the pandemic.

Additionally, SM has been valuable in recruiting hard-to-reach populations for research purposes. By using audience-specific strategies, researchers have been able to recruit participants quickly and with low cost. Despite questions related to data quality, this remains a promising way to recruit participants.[109]

Understanding Nuances of Different Types of Social Media Use

It will be an important task of future qualitative and quantitative research to more comprehensively assess content and contextual elements related to SM use. Much of the previous research has grouped multiple different ways of using SM together. By better understanding contextual factors associated with SM use, it will ultimately be easier to determine best practices for it.

Active versus passive social media use

Time on SM may be primarily spent viewing profiles, or it may be spent as an active participant, and these distinct patterns of use may have differential associations with mood conditions. Those who primarily observe are sometimes called "lurkers." It may be that those who are more active users feel more engaged and derive more sense of social capital from SM interactions. However, it also may be that active users are more prone to having negative exposures, which can affect self-cognitions.

One study found that active users of SM had 15% lower odds of depression, while passive users had 44% higher odds of depression. This study indicates that there is a difference in active versus passive SM use and how it affects mental health, but more information is needed to determine how much SM use impacts depression outcomes.[110]

Emotional valence of social media use

Additionally, it will be important to assess the overall emotional valence of SM interactions. Some individuals may primarily spend time "liking" others' posts, wishing friends happy birthday, and making positive comments. Others, however, may be prone to posting negative status updates or engaging in contentious interactions, which may be detrimental to relationship-building and lead to depression.[111]

Personality characteristics and social media use

People with different personality characteristics might have substantially different experiences with SM as it relates to mental disorders. For example, personality characteristics, such as extraversion, neuroticism, and openness, have been associated with increased online communication and SM use.[112,113] Therefore, it is possible that people with these characteristics might obtain more benefit from SM use. As a trait, extraversion is associated with high levels of engagement with the outside world, energy, and sociability, and this tendency may carry into the world of SM. Neuroticism is associated with anxiety, negative affect, and self-consciousness, all of which may also impact how individuals interact in a context related to SM. Conscientiousness is associated with organization, diligence, and impulse control. These qualities similarly may be relevant to how an individual approaches social interaction online. Finally, agreeableness is associated with altruism, consideration, and caring for others, all of which may be relevant to how individuals interact in SM-related situations. It would be valuable to more systematically assess how SM and personality characteristics interact so as to develop targeted interventions and recommendations.

Online and offline use

It would be valuable for future work to more comprehensively address associations between online and offline use. Some previous research studies have suggested that there may be a substitution effect; those who commit more time and attention to online activities may subsequently develop fewer close and meaningful offline relationships.[78,79] However, other studies suggest that those with increased online activities did not have any decrease in the quality of offline relationships.[114] Therefore, these will be important areas for further research. Ultimately, for example, it would be useful to know under what circumstances online interactions may be leveraged to improve offline support. This is especially true because individuals living with mental disorders may find it relatively easy to begin to engage in the online milieu, even when they have anhedonia, lack of energy, anxiety, and/or other symptoms preventing them from immediately engaging with the "real" world. This research is also important to help us in better understanding how to generate support for TAY with regard to relationship development. For example, among young adults aged 18 to 24 years and 25 to 34 years, 27% and 22% reported to use online dating sites to find potential sentimental partners, respectively, which represents a threefold increase from 2013.[115]

Use of multiple platforms

Associations between SM use and self-reported depression and anxiety may also be related to the use of multiple SM platforms. The number of different SM platforms used is rising substantially. On the one hand, increased use of multiple platforms may be associated with an increase in one's social capital and social support, which subsequently may be related to improvement of depression and anxiety symptoms.[116] However, use of multiple platforms also may involve multitasking, which as noted previously has been associated in the past with negative cognitive and mental health outcomes. Use of multiple SM platforms may also be related to negative mental health outcomes even if the different platforms are not all used at once. For example, the use of multiple platforms can lead to identity diffusion, which has been related to poor emotional health in the past.[117] This may be related to additional opportunities for online misunderstandings, negative interactions, and/or feelings of being left out, each of which may be associated with negative mood states.[118]

Balance of Risks and Opportunities for Use of Social Media in Treatment of Mental Health Conditions

There are both potential benefits and risks around using SM in the treatment of mental health conditions. Identified benefits include the ability to form therapeutic relationships even when there are barriers to seeking care, such as stigma, finances, or logistics. However, patient–provider relationships formed over SM may be inferior to those developed in person. Therefore, an important task of future research will be to determine under what circumstances and for whom SM-mediated mental health care is most valuable. For example, it may be useful to leverage SM in cases in which the barriers to in-person care are particularly profound. Similarly, there may be a role for the use of SM in the prevention of relapse. For example, SM could be leveraged to include medication reminders.

SUMMARY

In summary, SM has rapidly become an integral component of how transitional-age individuals connect with others. This has increased exponentially with the onset of the COVID-19 pandemic. Although literature around the influence of SM on development is still emerging, SM may facilitate a unique type of peer pressure through quantifiable social endorsement. There are potential benefits of using SM to alleviate mental health concerns, such as facilitation of connecting individuals with conditions such as depression, anxiety, and schizophrenia. Also, SM may be leveraged to provide mental health care and surveillance of mental health concerns. However, large cross-sectional epidemiologic studies suggest that increased SM use is linearly associated with prevalence of mental health concerns, such as depression, anxiety, and sleep disturbance. Future research should help to examine directionality of these associations and the role of contextual factors, such as style of SM use, personality, and the use of multiple platforms.

DISCLOSURE

The authors have nothing to disclose.

REFERENCES

1. Kaplan AM, Haenlein M. Users of the world, unite! the challenges and opportunities of social media. Bus Horiz 2010;53(1):59–68.
2. Statista. Social media usage in the United States - statistics & facts. 2021. Available at: https://www.statista.com/topics/3196/social-media-usage-in-the-united-states. Accessed July 13, 2021.
3. Pew Research Center. Social media use in 2021. 2021. Available at: https://www.pewresearch.org/internet/2021/04/07/social-media-use-in-2021. Accessed July 13, 2021.
4. Roisman GI, Masten AS, Coatsworth JD, et al. Salient and emerging developmental tasks in the transition to adulthood. Child Dev 2004;75:123–33.
5. Chou HTG, Edge N. "They are happier and having better lives than I am": the impact of using Facebook on perceptions of others' lives. Cyberpsychol Behav Soc Netw 2012;15(2):117–21.
6. Jelenchick LA, Eickhoff JC, Moreno MA. "Facebook depression?" Social networking site use and depression in older adolescents. J Adolesc Health 2013;52(1):128–30.
7. Statista. Most popular social networks worldwide as of January 2021, ranked by number of active users. 2021. Available at: https://www.statista.com/statistics/272014/global-social-networks-ranked-by-number-of-users. Accessed July 13, 2021.
8. Pantic I. Online social networking and mental health. Cyberpsychol Behav Soc Netw 2014;17(10):652–7.
9. Statista. Daily time spent on social networking by internet users worldwide from 2012 to 2020. 2021. Available at: https://www.statista.com/statistics/433871/daily-social-media-usage-worldwide. Accessed July 13, 2021.
10. Molla R. Posting less, posting more, and tired of it all: how the pandemic has changed social media. Vox; 2021. Available at: https://www.vox.com/recode/22295131/social-media-use-pandemic-covid-19-instagram-tiktok. Accessed July 13, 2021.
11. Zhou SJ, Zhang LG, Wang LL, et al. Prevalence of socio-demographic correlates of psychological health problems in Chinese adolescents during the outbreak of COVID-19. Euro Child Adol Psychiatry 2020;29(6):749–58.
12. Keles B, McCrae N, Grealish A. A systematic review: the influence of social media on depression, anxiety, and psychological distress in adolescents. Intl Journ of Adol and Youth 2020;25(1):79–93.
13. Wang G, Zhang Y, Zhao J, et al. Mitigate the effects of home confinement on children during the COVID-19 outbreak. Lancet 2020;395(10228):945–7.
14. Meshi D, Tamir DI, Heekeren HR. The emerging neuroscience of social media. Trends Cogn Sci 2015;19(12):771–82.

15. Ivie EJ, Pettitt A, Moses LJ, et al. A meta-analysis of the association between adolescent social media use and depressive symptoms. J Affect Disord 2020; 275:165–74.
16. Sherman LE, Payton AA, Hernandez LM, et al. The power of the like in adolescence: effects of peer influence on neural and behavioral responses to social media. Psychol Sci 2016;27(7):1027–35.
17. Choudhury S, McKinney KA. Digital media, the developing brain and the interpretive plasticity of neuroplasticity. Transcult Psychiatry 2013;50(2):192–215.
18. Ophir E, Nass C, Wagner AD. Cognitive control in media multitaskers. Proc Natl Acad Sci U S A 2009;106(37):15583–7.
19. Chen Q, Yan Z. Does multitasking with mobile phones affect learning? A review. Comput Hum Behav 2016;54:34–42.
20. Kiisel T. Is social media shortening our attention span? Forbes/Technology. 2012. Available at: http://www.forbes.com/sites/tykiisel/2012/01/25/is-social-media- shortening-our-attention-span/#4bfb2b486945. Accessed July 13, 2021.
21. Litsa T. How social media affects your attention span. Mountain View (CA): Linkedin; 2014. Available at: https://www.linkedin.com/pulse/20140519183028-114333012-how-social-media-affects-your-attention-span/. Accessed July 13, 2021.
22. Junco R, Cotten SR. The relationship between multitasking and academic performance. Comput Educ 2012;58(1):505–14.
23. Cain MS, Leonard JA, Gabrieli JDE, et al. Media multitasking in adolescence. Psychon Bull Rev 2016;23(6):1932–41.
24. Rosen L, Carrier LM, Cheever NA. Facebook and texting made me do it: media-induced task-switching while studying. Comput Hum Behav 2013;29:948–58.
25. van der Schuur WA, Baumgartner SE, Sumter SR, et al. The consequences of media multitasking for youth: a review. Comput Hum Behav 2015;53:204–15.
26. Becker MW, Alzahabi R, Hopwood CJ. Media multitasking is associated with symptoms of depression and social anxiety. Cyberpsychol Behav Soc Netw 2013;16(2):132–5.
27. Richards D, Caldwell PHY, Go H. Impact of social media on the health of children and young people. J Paediatr Child Health 2015;51(12):1152–7.
28. Shensa A, Sidani JE, Lin LY, et al. Social media use and perceived emotional support among US young adults. J Community Health 2016;41(3):541–9.
29. Mathiak K, Weber R. Toward brain correlates of natural behavior: fMRI during violent video games. Hum Brain Mapp 2006;27(12):948–56.
30. Guinta MR, John RM. Social media and adolescent health. Pediatr Nurs 2018; 44(4):196–201.
31. Bavelier D, Green CS, Dye MWG. Children, wired: for better and for worse. Neuron 2010;67(5):692–701.
32. Jashinsky J, Burton SH, Hanson CL, et al. Tracking suicide risk factors through Twitter in the US. Crisis 2013;35(1):51–9.
33. Larsen ME, Boonstra TW, Batterham PJ, et al. We feel: mapping emotion on twitter. IEEE J Biomed Heal Inform 2015;19(4):1246–52.
34. Sueki H. The association of suicide-related Twitter use with suicidal behaviour: a cross-sectional study of young Internet users in Japan. J Affect Disord 2015; 170:155–60.
35. McManus K, Mallory EK, Goldfeder RL, et al. Mining Twitter data to improve detection of schizophrenia. AMIA Jt Summits Transl Sci Proc 2015;2015:122–6.
36. Centers for Medicare & Medicaid Services. Centers for Medicare & Medicaid servics (CMS) and substance Abuse and mental health services administration

(SAMHSA): leveraging existing health and disease management programs to provide mental health and substance use disorder resources during the COVID-19 public health emergency (PHE). 2020. Available at: https://www.cms.gov/CCIIO/Programs-and-Initiatives/Health-Insurance-Marketplaces/Downloads/Mental-Health-Substance-Use-Disorder-Resources-COVID-19.pdf. Accessed July 13, 2021.

37. American Psychiatric Association. Practice guidance for COVID-19. 2020. Available at: https://www.psychiatry.org/psychiatrists/covid-19-coronavirus/practice-guidance-for-covid-19. Accessed July 13, 2021.

38. Di Carlo F, Sociali A, Picutti E, et al. Telepsychiatry and other cutting-edge technologies in COVID-19 pandemic: bridging the distance in mental health assistance. Int J Clin Pract 2021;75(1):e13716.

39. Cox-George C. The changing face(book) of psychiatry: can we justify "following" patients' social media activity? Bjpsych Bull 2015;39(6):283–4.

40. Välimaki M, Athanasopoulou C, Lahti M, et al. Effectiveness of social media interventions for people with schizophrenia: a systematic review and meta-analysis. J Med Internet Res 2016;18(4):e92.

41. Merolli M, Gray K, Martin-Sanchez F. Health outcomes and related effects of using social media in chronic disease management: a literature review and analysis of affordances. J Biomed Inform 2013;46(6):957–69.

42. Merolli M, Gray K, Martin-Sanchez F. Therapeutic affordances of social media: emergent themes from a global online survey of people with chronic pain. J Med Internet Res 2014;16(12):e284.

43. Evans WD. Social marketing campaigns and children's media use. Future Child 2008;18(1):181–203.

44. Kuo MH, Orsmond GI, Coster WJ, et al. Media use among adolescents with autism spectrum disorder. Autism 2014;18:914–23.

45. Dosani S, Harding C, Wilson S. Online groups and patient forums. Curr Psychiatry Rep 2014;16(11):507.

46. National Alliance on Mental Illness (NAMI). Support & education. 2021. Available at: https://nami.org/Support-Education. Accessed July 13, 2021.

47. Szlyk H, Deng J, Xu C, et al. Leveraging social media to explore the barriers to treatment among individuals with depressive symptoms. Depress Anxiety 2020;37(5):458–65.

48. Ridout B, Campbell A. The use of social networking sites in mental health interventions for young people: systematic review. J Med Internet Res 2018;20(12):e12244.

49. Kata A. Anti-vaccine activists, Web 2.0, and the postmodern paradigm - an overview of tactics and tropes used online by the anti-vaccination movement. Vaccine 2012;30(25):3778–89.

50. Moreno MA, Jelenchick LA, Egan KG, et al. Feeling bad on Facebook: depression disclosures by college students on a social networking site. Depress Anxiety 2011;28(6):447–55.

51. Whitehill J, Brockman L, Moreno M. "Just talk to me": communicating with college students about depression disclosures on Facebook. J Adolesc Health 2013;52(1):122–7.

52. De Choudhury M, De S. Mental health discourse on Reddit: self-disclosure, social support, and anonymity. Proc Eight Int AAAI Conf Weblogs Soc Media held at Ann Arbor, MI, May 27–29, 2015.

53. Naslund JA, Aschbrenner KA, Marsch LA, et al. The future of mental health care: peer-to-peer support and social media. Epidemiol Psychiatr Sci 2016;25(2): 113–22.
54. Betton V, Borschmann R, Docherty M, et al. The role of social media in reducing stigma and discrimination. Br J Psychiatry 2015;206(6):443–4.
55. Shensa A, Sidani JE, Escobar-Viera CG, et al. Emotional support from social media and face-to-face relationships: associations with depression risk among young adults. J Affect Disord 2020;260:38–44.
56. Shensa A, Sidani JE, Escobar-Viera CG, et al. Real-life closeness of social media contacts and depressive symptoms among university students. J Am Coll Health 2018;66(8):747–53.
57. Digrazia J, McKelvey K, Bollen J, et al. More tweets, more votes: social media as a quantitative indicator of political behavior. PLoS One 2013;8(11):e79449.
58. Doan S, Vo B, Collier N. An analysis of Twitter messages in the 2011 Tohoku earthquake. In: Kostkova P, Szomszor M, Fowler D, editors. Electronic healthcare: fourth international conference, eHealth 2011. Lecture notes of the institute for computer sciences, social informatics and telecommunications engineering, vol. 91. Berlin: Springer; 2012. p. 58–66.
59. Broniatowski DA, Paul MJ, Dredze M. National and local influenza surveillance through twitter: an analysis of the 2012-2013 influenza epidemic. PLoS One 2013;8(12):e83672.
60. Collier N, Son NT, Nguyen NM. OMG u got flu? Analysis of shared health messages for bio-surveillance. J Biomed Semantics 2011;2(Suppl 5):S9.
61. St Louis C, Zorlu G. Can Twitter predict disease outbreaks? Br Med J 2012;344: e2353.
62. Haas A, Koestner B, Rosenberg J, et al. An interactive web-based method of outreach to college students at risk for suicide. J Am Coll Health 2008;57(1): 15–22.
63. Won H, Myung W, Song G, et al. Predicting national suicide numbers with social media data. PLoS One 2013;8(4):e61809.
64. Robinson J, Cox G, Bailey E, et al. Social media and suicide prevention: a systematic review. Early Interv Psychiatry 2016;10(2):103–21.
65. Mikal J, Hurst S, Conway M. Ethical issues in using Twitter for population-level depression monitoring: a qualitative study. BMC Med Ethics 2016;17:22.
66. Kim J, Uddin ZA, Lee Y, et al. A systematic review of the validity of screening depression through Facebook, twitter, Instagram, and Snapchat. J Affect Disord 2021;286:360–9.
67. Negriff S. Depressive symptoms predict characteristics of online social networks. J Adolesc Health 2019;65(1):101–6.
68. Kramer ADI, Guillory JE, Hancock JT. Experimental evidence of massive-scale emotional contagion through social networks. Proc Natl Acad Sci U S A 2014; 111(24):8788–90.
69. Lin R, Utz S. The emotional responses of browsing Facebook: happiness, envy, and the role of tie strength. Comput Hum Behav 2015;52:29–38.
70. Ellison NB, Steinfield C, Lampe C. The benefits of Facebook "friends": social capital and college students' use of online social network sites. J Comput Commun 2007;12(4):1143–68.
71. Valenzuela S, Park N, Kee KF. Is there social capital in a social network site? Facebook use and college students' life satisfaction, trust, and participation. J Comput Commun 2009;14(4):875–901.

72. de la Pena A, Quintanilla C. Share, like and achieve: the power of Facebook to reach health-related goals. Int J Consum Stud 2015;39(5):495–505.

73. Bessiere K, Pressman S, Kiesler S, et al. Effects of Internet use on health and depression: a longitudinal study. J Med Internet Res 2010;12(1):e6.

74. Lin LY, Sidani JE, Shensa A, et al. Association between social media use and depression among U.S. young adults. Depress Anxiety 2016;33(4):323–31.

75. Naja WJ, Kansoun AH, Haddad RS. Prevalence of depression in medical students at the Lebanese university and exploring its correlation with Facebook relevance: a questionnaire study. JMIR Res Protoc 2016;5(2):e96.

76. Woods HC, Scott H. #Sleepyteens: social media use in adolescence is associated with poor sleep quality, anxiety, depression and low self-esteem. J Adolesc 2016;51:41–9.

77. Marar Z. Intimacy: understanding the subtle power of human connection. Durham (United Kingdom): Acumen Publishing; 2012.

78. Baek YM, Bae Y, Jang H. Social and parasocial relationships on social network sites and their differential relationships with users' psychological well-being. Cyberpsychol Behav Soc Netw 2013;16(7):512–7.

79. Primack BA, Shensa A, Sidani JE, et al. Temporal associations between social media use and depression. Am J Prev Med 2021;60(2):179–88.

80. Primack BA, Bisbey MA, Shensa A, et al. The association between valence of social media experiences and depressive symptoms. Depress Anxiety 2018;35(8):784–94.

81. Jeri-Yabar A, Sanchez-Carbonel A, Tito K, et al. Association between social media use (Twitter, Instagram, Facebook) and depressive symptoms: are Twitter users at higher risk? Int J Soc Psychiatry 2019;65(1):14–9.

82. Dyson MP, Hartling L, Shulhan J, et al. A systematic review of social media use to discuss and view deliberate self-harm acts. PLoS One 2016;11(5):e0155813.

83. Escobar-Viera CG, Whitfield DL, Wessel CB, et al. For better or for worse? A systematic review of the evidence on social media use and depression among lesbian, gay, and bisexual minorities. JMIR Ment Health 2018;5(3):e10496.

84. Cunningham S, Hudson CC, Harkness K. Social media and depression symptoms: a meta-analysis. Res Child Adolesc Psychopathol 2021;49:241–53.

85. Schou Andreassen C, Billieux J, Griffiths MD, et al. The relationship between addictive use of social media and video games and symptoms of psychiatric disorders: a large-scale cross-sectional study. Psychol Addict Behav 2016;30(2):252–62.

86. Lee-Won RJ, Herzog L, Park SG. Hooked on Facebook: the role of social anxiety and need for social assurance in problematic use of Facebook. Cyberpsychol Behav Soc Netw 2015;18(10):567–74.

87. Levenson JC, Shensa A, Sidani JE, et al. The association between social media use and sleep disturbance among young adults. Prev Med 2016;85:36–41.

88. Royant-Parola S, Londe V, Tréhout S, et al. Nouveaux médias sociaux, nouveaux comportements de sommeil chez les adolescents [The use of social media modifies teenagers' sleep-related behavior]. Encephale 2018;44(4):321–8. French.

89. Oksanen A, Garcia D, Rasanen P. Proanorexia communities on social media. Pediatrics 2016;137(1).

90. Oksanen A, Garcia D, Sirola A, et al. Pro-anorexia and anti-pro-anorexia videos on YouTube: sentiment analysis of user responses. J Med Internet Res 2015;17(11):e256.

91. Juarez L, Soto E, Pritchard ME. Drive for muscularity and drive for thinness: the impact of pro-anorexia websites. Eat Disord 2012;20(2):99–112.

92. Sidani JE, Shensa A, Hoffman B, et al. The association between social media use and eating concerns among US young adults. J Acad Nutr Diet 2016;116(9):1465–72.

93. Mazurek MO, Shattuck PT, Wagner M, et al. Prevalence and correlates of screen-based media use among youths with autism spectrum disorders. J Autism Dev Disord 2012;42(8):1757–67.

94. Mazurek MO, Wenstrup C. Television, video game and social media use among children with ASD and typically developing siblings. J Autism Dev Disord 2013;43(6):1258–71.

95. Shane HC, Albert PD. Electronic screen media for persons with autism spectrum disorders: results of a survey. J Autism Dev Disord 2008;38(8):1499–508.

96. Kross E, Verduyn P, Demiralp E, et al. Facebook use predicts declines in subjective well-being in young adults. PLoS One 2013;8(8):e69841.

97. Caplan SE. Problematic Internet use and psychosocial well-being: development of a theory-based cognitive-behavioral measurement instrument. Comput Hum Behav 2002;18(5):553–75.

98. Sanders CE, Field TM, Diego M, et al. The relationship of Internet use to depression and social isolation among adolescents. Adolescence 2000;35(138):237–42.

99. Davis RA. Cognitive-behavioral model of pathological Internet use. Comput Hum Behav 2001;17(2):187–95.

100. Morahan-Martin J, Schumacher P. Loneliness and social uses of the Internet. Comput Hum Behav 2003;19(6):659–71.

101. Korkeila J. The relationships depression and Internet addiction. Duodecim 2012;128(7):741–8.

102. Sagioglou C, Greitemeyer T. Facebook's emotional consequences: why Facebook causes a decrease in mood and why people still use it. Comput Hum Behav 2014;35:359–63.

103. American College Health Association. American College Health AssociationNational College Health assessment II: reference group executive summary 2015. Hanover (MD): American College Health Association; 2016.

104. Block JJ. Issues for DSM-V: internet addiction. Am J Psychiatry 2008;165(3):306–7.

105. Morrison CM, Gore H. The relationship between excessive Internet use and depression: a questionnaire-based study of 1,319 young people and adults. Psychopathology 2010;43(2):121–6.

106. O'Keeffe GS, Clarke-Pearson K. The impact of social media on children, adolescents, and families. Pediatrics 2011;127(4):800–4.

107. Hill RM, Rufino K, Kurian S, et al. Suicide ideation and attempts in a pediatric emergency department before and during COVID-19. Pediatrics 2021;147(3). e2020029280.

108. Guillory J, Wiant KF, Farrelly M, et al. Recruiting hard-to-reach populations for survey research: using Facebook and Instagram advertisements and in-person Intercept in LGBT bars and nightclubs to recruit LGBT young adults. J Med Internet Res 2018;20(6):e197.

109. Escobar-Viera CG, Shensa A, Bowman ND, et al. Passive and active social media use and depressive symptoms among United States adults. Cyberpsychol Behav Soc Netw 2018;21(7):437–43.

110. Forest AL, Wood JV. When social networking is not working: individuals with low self-esteem recognize but do not reap the benefits of self-disclosure on Facebook. Psychol Sci 2012;23(3):295–302.

111. Mark G, Ganzach Y. Personality and Internet usage: a large-scale representative study of young adults. Comput Hum Behav 2014;36:274–81.

112. Correa T, Hinsley AW, de Zuniga HG. Who interacts on the Web? The intersection of users' personality and social media use. Comput Hum Behav 2010;26(2): 247–53.

113. Park J, Lee DS, Shablack H, et al. When perceptions defy reality: the relationships between depression and actual and perceived Facebook social support. J Affect Disord 2016;200:37–44.

114. Lenhart A, Duggan M. Couples, the Internet and social media. Washington, DC: Pew Res Cent; 2014. Available at: http://www.pewinternet.org/files/2014/02/PIP_Couples_and_Technology-FIN_021114.pdf. Accessed January 3, 2017.

115. Keitzmann JH, Hermkens K, McCarthy IP, et al. Social media? Get serious! Understanding the functional building blocks of social media. Bus Horiz 2011;54: 241–51.

116. Marcia JE. Identity in adolescence. In: Adelson J, editor. Handbook of adolescent psychology. New York: Wiley; 1980. p. 159–87.

117. Arnett JJ. Adolescents' uses of media for self-socialization. J Youth Adolesc 1995;24(5):519–33.

Mental Health Care of Detained Youth Within Juvenile Detention Facilities

Kevin Whitley, MD, MA[a], Camille Tastenhoye, MD[b],
Amanda Downey, MD[c], John S. Rozel, MD, MSL, DFAPA[d],*

KEYWORDS

- Mental health treatment • Juvenile justice • Juvenile detention
- Trauma-informed care • Solitary confinement • Isolation • Seclusion

KEY POINTS

- Youth in the juvenile justice system have a high prevalence of a diverse array of mental disorders and severe psychosocial stressors.
- Trauma is common, and trauma-informed care should be considered a universal precaution in working with justice-involved youth.
- Youth can benefit significantly from evidence-based psychosocial and pharmacologic interventions.
- Although clinically ordered and supervised seclusion may be appropriate in limited situations, disciplinary or punitive use of isolation or solitary confinement is categorically inappropriate.

INTRODUCTION

Mental health treatment of juvenile offenders and undocumented immigrant youth in detention provides a unique opportunity for treatment providers. Although the work may be challenging, the clinical needs and opportunities for early and meaningful interventions are significant. Adjudication "is the court process that determines (judges) if the juvenile committed the act for which he or she is charged. The term 'adjudicated' is analogous to 'convicted' and indicates that the court concluded the juvenile committed the act."[1] Common causes of youth adjudication include violence directed

[a] Southwood Psychiatric Hospital, 2575 Boyce Plaza Road, Pittsburgh, PA 15241, USA; [b] Department of Psychiatry, University of Pittsburgh School of Medicine, UPMC Western Psychiatric Hospital, 3811 O'Hara Street, Pittsburgh, PA 15213, USA; [c] Division of Adolescent and Young Adult Medicine, Department of Pediatrics, Department of Psychiatry and Behavioral Sciences, University of California, San Francisco, 3333 California Street, Suite 245, San Francisco, CA 94118, USA; [d] University of Pittsburgh, resolve Crisis Services of UPMC Western Psychiatric Hospital, 333 N Braddock Avenue, Pittsburgh, PA 15208, USA
* Corresponding author.
E-mail address: rozeljs@upmc.edu

Child Adolesc Psychiatric Clin N Am 31 (2022) 31–44
https://doi.org/10.1016/j.chc.2021.09.002
1056-4993/22/© 2021 Elsevier Inc. All rights reserved.
childpsych.theclinics.com

at others, vandalism, burglary or robbery, status offenses including curfew violation, loitering or disorderly conduct, truancy, running away, underage drinking, trespassing, weapons offenses, drug abuse violations, and driving under the influence. Less common reasons for adjudication include aggravated assault, homicide, manslaughter, arson, gambling, embezzlement, forgery, counterfeiting, prostitution, obstruction of justice, and sexual deviance.

Many reasons for the adjudication of youth exist. Often the youths' causes for adjudication are complex: comorbid psychosocial conditions and stressors are common. Youthful offenses are frequently influenced by poverty, disenfranchisement, poor access to jobs, residential segregation, schools ill-equipped to address acting-out behaviors, family structure including single-parent households and family disruption or a parent in prison, substance use, mental health disorders, and so forth. Community level structural factors impede systemic social organizations and often impede living within the constraints of the law.[2]

Mental health care of youth in the juvenile justice system and asylum-seeking youth in detention provides a unique opportunity to address and remedy social constraints in the context of psychiatric illness. Adjudicated youth and undocumented immigrant youth have significantly higher rates of mental illness than youth in the general population.[3] The prevalence of mental health disorders in adjudicated youth in nonresidential facilities is estimated to be 50%.[4] Asylum seeking youth were often exposed to violence and as a result seek residence in another country. The prevalence of mental illness among youth involved in the juvenile justice system located in residential treatment facilities is estimated to be between 65% and 70%.[4] Youth in the juvenile justice system can have any illness within the spectrum of mental illness. Behavioral disorders such as conduct disorder are the most frequently diagnosed mental illnesses in adjudicated youth at 62% for male youth and 48% for female youth.[4] Substance use disorders occur in 46.2% of adjudicated youth.[4] According to Wasserman and colleagues, anxiety disorders are estimated to affect 34.4% of youth in the juvenile justice system,[4] and 18.3% of adjudicated youth have mood disorders.[4] Reportedly, 10.6% of male youth and 29.2% of female youth have clinical depression.[5] Attention-deficit/hyperactivity disorder prevalence is measured at 21% for male youth and 24% for female youth.[5] In addition, it is estimated that up to 19% of detained youths are suicidal during detention, and approximately 50% of female youth in the juvenile justice system have symptoms of posttraumatic stress disorder (PTSD).[5] It is common for youth to have more than one mental disorder. When conduct disorder is removed as a possible mental disorder in adjudicated youth, 66.3% of youth meet criteria for a mental disorder.[6] The problems adjudicated children face are diverse. Each child's social and mental health needs are unique. Despite the heterogeneity of the problems faced by adjudicated youth, mental health treatment has been shown to reduce recidivism rates by 25% compared with children who are not treated for psychiatric illness.[7] The most successful programs have reduced recidivism rates by 25% to 80%.[8]

PRINCIPLES OF ADJUDICATED YOUTH MENTAL HEALTH TREATMENT

When possible, diversion to community-based, integrated mental health services is preferable to incarceration. When these less-restrictive resources have been exhausted and adjudication and further juvenile justice involvement is mandatory, youth should have access to evidence-based medical treatments.[9,10] Although involvement in juvenile court may grant access to mental and physical health treatment, social services, family-based services, and educational services that would otherwise not be available, entrance to the juvenile justice system should not be motivated by increasing access to these services. Entry into the juvenile court system itself may exacerbate underlying mental health conditions due to overcrowding, lack of appropriate treatment, restrictive housing, separation from support systems, and other potential traumas.[9]

Services provided by the juvenile justice system should be child and family focused, culturally competent, and developmentally appropriate. Mental health services should be equipped to respond to issues of gender, ethnicity, race, age, sexual orientation, socioeconomic status, and faith.[11] When possible, families should be made active participants in their child's mental health treatment. Families who are equipped with information about the process of justice involvement and treatment can serve as strong advocates and support systems for their child while navigating these systems.[11] Mental health treatment providers should ideally collaborate with all systems of care to create a unique and individualized treatment approach. Equally important is the training of law enforcement and juvenile justice staff to interact with youth with behavioral health conditions in a way that is trauma informed and strengths based.[11]

The National Mental Health Association identified a series of values and principles inherent to the care of children in the juvenile justice system in the publication *Mental Health Treatment for Youth in the Juvenile Justice System: A Compendium of Promising Practices* (2004):[12]

- Early identification and intervention are vital to promoting positive outcomes. Children must have access to a comprehensive array of individualized formal and informal services that address their physical, emotional, social, and educational needs. Services should be delivered in the least restrictive, normative environment that is clinically appropriate.
- Families and caregivers should be full participants in all aspects of policy development and the planning and delivery of services, which should be integrated with linkages between child and family serving agencies and programs.
- Care coordination should be provided to ensure that multiple services are linked and clinically indicated. They should also address a family's strengths and needs and be reviewed on a regular basis for applicability to the family's current level of functioning.
- The service delivery system should include providers who help enable smooth transitions to adult services, if necessary.
- The rights of children should be protected and effective advocacy efforts should be promoted.
- Services must be provided without regard to race, religion, national origin, sex, physical disability, or similar characteristics.

Recent changes in the juvenile justice system emphasize a public health–based model of care that is a more rehabilitative and strengths-based model in which youth are viewed as having the potential for positive growth.[9] The needs of justice-involved youth and their families are complex and cannot be adequately addressed by one universal approach. Done well, comprehensive and collaborative mental health services within the juvenile justice system reduce recidivism and lead to decreased future juvenile justice involvement, with the hope of positively affecting individual and family functioning.[12]

TRAUMA ISSUES IN JUVENILE JUSTICE

Numerous studies have identified high rates of PTSD and trauma in adjudicated youth, with trauma history considered a risk factor for eventual involvement in the juvenile court system.[13,14] Sexual trauma is considered a major risk factor for female youth, particularly female youth of color.[15] Trauma may include experiences while in placement or foster care, including physical or sexual assault or witnessing the assault of other youth, as well as traumatic losses and victimization in the community. Repeated traumatization is common, and one study identified that 5% of incarcerated youth have had 11 or more major traumatic experiences.[14] "Complex trauma," referring to exposure to traumatic stressors that compromises secure attachment and the ability to self-regulate emotions, is common among incarcerated youth.[16] Complex, chronic, and early childhood traumas can also have profound impacts on subsequent neurodevelopment and functioning.[17,18]

Trauma-related symptoms may be misinterpreted as symptoms in need of disciplinary intervention by criminal justice professionals. For example, exaggerated startle responses may be construed as aggression, and dissociative freezing may be seen as noncompliance.

Trauma-focused treatment is generally recognized to be most effective when it occurs in a stable, safe therapeutic setting.[19,20] Effective treatment of trauma involves medications and psychotherapy and should occur in the context of a therapeutic relationship that is stable and experienced as safe for the consumer. One of the most significant limitations of trauma work in juvenile justice settings is the stability of the therapeutic relationship. A therapeutic context is more challenging to achieve in many juvenile justice settings, often jeopardized by lack of clinical control over length of treatment or the environment of care. The therapeutic relationship may be further challenged by the youth's reluctance to disclose traumatic experiences involving criminal conduct of the youth or others.[21]

CRISIS MANAGEMENT OF YOUTH IN DETENTION CENTERS

In addition to all of the intrinsic psychosocial risk factors that justice-involved youth live with (and which may well have predisposed them to justice involvement), the detention process itself can be stressful. Detention centers need to be able to balance facility security needs with compassionate, calming interventions that can deescalate youth and support them through the criminal justice process. Even for a youth with a relatively pristine prior mental health history and substantial social supports, the process of detention and proceeding through the justice process can be extremely distressing. Finally, failure to adequately manage underlying psychiatric disorders (eg, ongoing medication management, coordination with other treatment providers) can lead to acute decompensation as well.

Newly detained youth may be apprehensive about the new setting and may have acute psychosocial stressors. Further, suicidal thoughts, recent suicidal behavior, and current passive death wish or hopelessness are common in incarcerated youth and are spontaneously reported only half of the time.[22]

When adapting clinical strategies for agitation and acute crisis management to juvenile justice settings care must be taken. Fundamental strategies such as deescalation and consideration of underlying medical and psychiatric contributions to agitation remain critical.[23–25] However, clinicians need to recognize that justice setting may lack common safeguards that are used in managing agitation in clinical settings, including availability of a nurse to monitor vital signs or medical issues, routine observation during seclusion, justifications for initiating and ending physical interventions, or even the simple matter of notifying the psychiatrist of the incident. Establishing clear policies in alignment with clinical ethics and standards from groups such as the National Council for Correctional Health Care is important. Strategically, and with any intervention for agitation, underlying causes need to be addressed. Biological interventions—and for that matter, restraints and holds—will do little to mitigate underlying contextual stressors and contributors to crisis and agitation.[25]

Intake processes should include steps to identify prior psychiatric history as well as routine screening to identify previously unrecognized pathology. Adequate and ongoing training and supervision of staff for recognizing and managing distress and agitation—with an emphasis on promoting prevention and verbal deescalation over physical interventions—should be supported. Whenever possible, evaluation, screening, and supportive interventions should occur routinely and as early as possible in the detention process: it is much safer for youth and staff alike to prevent crises than to respond to them.

Notably, improved management of behavioral crises in the community may play a critical role in reducing entry into the criminal justice system. There has been increased recognition of the impact of systemic bias, police response to behavioral emergencies, and criminalization of psychosocial illness and crisis.[26] Joint law enforcement/behavioral health community crisis response teams have existed for 30 years.[27] There is growing evidence that they improve the ability to divert people with primarily mental health concerns out of the criminal justice system.[28]

TREATMENT OF DISRUPTIVE, IMPULSE CONTROL, AND CONDUCT-RELATED DISORDER IN DELINQUENT YOUTH

Disruptive, impulse control, and conduct-related disorders are of particular concern in juvenile justice settings. Almost by definition, most youth entering the juvenile justice system have some pattern of behavior that threatens the physical, financial, or emotional welfare of others. It is common for youth to enter the legal system after committing acts of battery, assault, vandalism, or other acts that jeopardize the rights of others. If there is a pattern of aggressive, deceitful, dangerous, or difficult behavior that violates social norms and creates conflict with individuals in a position of authority, a diagnosis of disruptive, impulse control, and conduct disorder should be considered.[29]

Treating disruptive, impulse control, and conduct disorders often proves challenging. Research shows that children with significant disruptive behavior benefit from skills-based interventions[30]; parenting/teacher skills training; individual, family based, and group therapy; and behavioral therapy to improve peer interactions and compliance with requests from authority figures.[31] Multisystemic therapy and behavioral therapy should focus on problem-solving skills and social competence through the utilization of community supports and positive community and family attributes.[32] When family involvement in treatment is not an option, youth require enhanced social skill training, which includes social skills acquisition, vocational training, academic assistance and direction, and life skills acquisition.[32]

Any youth who is noncompliant with treatment and repeatedly places others at risk of harm, even if the risk of harm is mild, should be considered for treatment in a residential treatment facility. Adequate residential facility treatment entails a multiple-phase program. Successful residential treatment programs are often cognitive behavior therapy focused and include, but are not limited to, (1) social skill training, (2) anger management, and (3) moral reasoning. Each phase is multipronged. The programs average around 10 weeks in duration but can take up to 2 years to complete, especially if the child has a severe pattern of conduct disorder behavior or low intelligence quotient.

In addition to behavioral therapy, family therapy, and treatment in a residential treatment facility, there is evidence that medications improve symptoms of disruptive, impulse control, and conduct disorders.[33] At present there are no US Food and Drug Administration–approved medications to help guide treatment in this population.

There can be several barriers to "ideal" clinical care for adjudicated youth. In an ideal world, for example, a child psychiatrist can match evidence-based treatments to clear diagnoses with minimal comorbidity established by extended evaluation and adequate collateral and follow the patient over an extended, longitudinal course. Youth involved in the justice system, however, are marked by a convergence of risk factors and complicating issues: comorbidity is high, courses of treatment interrupted and fractured, psychosocial and historical risk factors prominent, and collateral often lacking. They are embedded in a system where, as so much else, race seems to determine many factors including diagnosis.[34] Further, the active family involvement that can be critical in the care of any psychiatrically ill youth is often impaired—either by the prominent psychosocial stressors affecting the families themselves or the pattern of repeated placements away from the family. Finally, youth and informants may have any number of different motivations to exaggerate, minimize, or fabricate symptoms as explanations for criminal behavior, justifications for shifting the level of care, or simply to obtain medications for their sedating or stimulating effects.

Although therapy may be a treatment of choice for many mental health disorders, adjudicated youth are often transient, presenting challenges for treatments requiring multiple sessions. For some adjudicated youth, consistent therapy is not an option and medication management may be easier to sustain than consistent talk therapy, although entering either course of treatment is fraught with some degree of risk. Several issues may be considered when deciding on medication management in this context (**Box 1**). State laws vary significantly on rules for consent to medication treatment of minors, and some states make additional qualifications for medication treatment of youth in juvenile justice settings.[35]

SECLUSION, ISOLATION, AND SOLITARY CONFINEMENT

Although seclusion and isolation may seem as similar concepts, they have distinct meanings in the context of juvenile correctional care. Seclusion and restraint are clinical interventions; isolation and solitary confinement are disciplinary measures. The National Commission on Correctional Health Care permits clinically indicated seclusion or restraint within narrow parameters but no longer allows isolation or solitary confinement.[36]

Box 1
Issues considered by prescribers before initiating or adjusting medication in adjudicated youth

- How certain is the diagnosis?

- How good is the evidence for a given medication for that diagnosis? Is the youth willing to continue to take the medication, even across placements? Are the parents or legal guardians in agreement with medication? What are the legal parameters for consent, given the age of the patient and the patient's legal status?

- Are there significant risks if the medication is suddenly discontinued due to a poor transition in care between placements or going on the run?

- If a medication is being added, changed, or removed, is the psychiatrist reasonably likely to have an adequate opportunity to monitor the patient for the effect of those changes?

In short, what are the risks of treatment and nontreatment in a correct-diagnosis or an incorrect-diagnosis scenario?

Seclusion is the use of a separate physical space for a youth because of acute psychiatric symptoms that cannot be otherwise controlled through less restrictive means and serves as a therapeutic intervention at the direction of a physician in response to psychiatric symptoms creating imminent danger to a patient or to others. The purpose of seclusion is management of agitation and prevention of harm. Seclusion is time limited and is monitored, initiated, and ended based on clinical criteria and real-time assessment. Seclusion and therapeutic physical holds may be clinically and ethically appropriate in some limited situations in juvenile justice settings.

In contrast, isolation and solitary confinement are disciplinary interventions that are intended to be punitive or used to address security concerns. Isolation and solitary confinement generally allow little to no contact with any people except for facility staff and are not seen as being therapeutic. Such conditions can be very harmful to the well-being of the isolated person and raise significant ethical concerns. The American Academy of Child and Adolescent Psychiatry issued a policy statement in 2012 that permits the use of therapeutic seclusion in accordance with relevant laws and regulations but strongly discourages the use of solitary confinement or isolation and categorically disapproves of any seclusion or isolation greater than 24 hours.[37] Guidance on prohibited practices relating to isolation and solitary confinement for juveniles is an ongoing project of the American Civil Liberties Union (extensive resources available at <u>https://www.aclu.org/report/alone-afraid</u>). Any use of seclusion, restraint, isolation, or solitary confinement should occur in accordance with written and reviewed policies maintained by the facility and that are in alignment with relevant federal and state regulations, laws, and ethical standards.

Insofar as appropriate clinical, regulatory, and policy standards are followed, use of clinical seclusion and restraint may be appropriate in some circumstances. However, clinicians should be mindful that they may be asked to support or condone the correctional staff's use of isolation or other punitive or security interventions even when those interventions are clearly not clinically driven. In addition, there are, inevitably, many cases that are complex and ambiguous. Clinicians are encouraged to seek consultation for any ethically challenging decision and avoid lending support to questionable practices. New resources from national professional associations have recently been released to mitigate the use of seclusion and isolation in juvenile justice settings.[38]

Seclusion Considerations in the Setting of Covid-19

In spring 2020, the coronavirus-19 was declared a global pandemic by the Centers for Disease Control and Prevention. In the months following, juvenile correctional facilities began using isolation as a health precaution, given the difficulties of maintaining social distancing in facilities.[39] Although the use of isolation is nonpunitive, the literature has equated isolation for the purposes of health precautions to solitary confinement. Solitary confinement is known to have psychological effects on youth, including worsened depression, anger, obsessive thoughts, paranoia and psychosis, and elevated risk of suicide.[39] This isolation has been exacerbated by restrictions on in-person visits, both within the facilities themselves as well as with regard to interstate travel. There is no literature available at this time regarding the effects of the pandemic on the overall physical and mental health of adjudicated youth, as it relates to isolation and confinement.

DISCRIMINATION, MENTAL HEALTH, AND ADJUDICATED YOUTH

Racism is a complicated and common problem within society. Because of police brutality toward black individuals and the overrepresentation of minorities in the legal system in the United States the American Psychological Association (APA) classified racism as a pandemic. Research has repeatedly documented racial disparities in the health care and the legal system. The consequences of racism and sexism affect the health status of children, adolescents, and their families not only in general but also in detained youth. Implicit and explicit racial and sexual biases influence acute stress, anxiety, PTSD, compulsive behaviors, obsessive thinking, low self-esteem, truancy, increase in high school dropout rates, somatic complaints, heart disease, obesity, diabetes, hypertension, and generalized poor physical and mental health.[40] Research also indicates minorities are less likely to seek mental health services due to perceived biases by health care providers, negative experiences during mental health treatment, and discriminatory practices by health care providers.[40]

The juvenile detention system is not immune to racial and sexual discrimination. Two examples of discrimination in the juvenile detention system include the overrepresentation of black youth placed in solitary confinement and the overcriminalization of lesbian, gay, bisexual, and transgendered youth. Race has a prominent role in the discretionary decision to place minority adolescents in solitary confinement. Black youth have a 68.8% greater odds of placement in solitary confinement in juvenile detention than youth of other races after controlling for variables.[41] LGBT adolescents experience higher rates of adjudication and detention for nonviolent crimes than any other demographic of youth.[42]

Resolving discriminatory practices within juvenile detention and health care is complicated. To adequately address prejudice in juvenile detention, treatment providers and institutions must recognize their own biases and discriminatory practices. For example, an inpatient child and adolescent hospital may place black youth with older children due to false perceptions of violence or age. Institutional leaders must proactively seek methods to improve mental health care by providing professional education at the institutional and individual level that addresses racial disparity. Individual treatment providers must recognize racial prejudices and actively address the potential consequences. In order to address racial disparity within mental health the APA and National Alliance for Mental Illness recommends the following:

- Include culturally competent services that recognize traditions, histories, values, and beliefs.
- Address minority patients' preferences. Sensitivity and responsiveness to the child or adolescents needs requires ascertaining what matters to the patient and acknowledging the patient's experiences.
- The system can support providers with shared decision-making and improved communication skills and interpersonal relationships through education.
- Ask the patient about their preferences and practice active listening with follow-up questions.
- Recognize the impact of the community on the patient including mental health symptoms.
- Improve evidence-based practices through research.

INTEGRATED CARE IN JUVENILE DETENTION

Unmet physical health needs among youth in the juvenile correctional system are a crucial point of intervention. According to the Survey of Youth in Residential Placement, more than two-thirds of youth identified a health care need, including injury, problems with vision or hearing, dental needs, or "other illness."[43] Pediatricians and other health care providers deliver care to this high-risk population, particularly in the arena of dental care, traumatic injury, tuberculosis, sexually transmitted infections, and pregnancy.[43,44] According to the National Commission on Correctional

Healthcare's *Standards for Health Services in Juvenile Detention and Confinement Facilities*, youth should be screened on arrival for urgent health care or mental health needs, followed by a comprehensive health and mental health screening. A policy statement by the American Academy of Pediatrics (AAP) for Health Care for Youth in the Juvenile Justice System calls for delivery of the same level and standards of medical and mental health care as nonincarcerated use in their communities.[44] Although some service delivery may be mitigated by length of stay in the facility, at minimum, care should include the identification and treatment of immediate medical and psychiatric needs. Close coordination and collaboration between mental health and medical providers can help ensure all needs are adequately addressed, as well as to ensure continuity of care and prevention of duplicate services. All providers can help youth and families identify a medical home within the community and collaborate with probation officers who often help families navigate medical and mental health care follow-up on reentry into the community.[44]

Working with Families of Justice Involved

Family plays an integral part in the positive and negative outcomes of adjudicated youth in and out of juvenile detention facilities. Positive family involvement provides a supportive and emotionally stable environment in addition to the navigation of the needs of the child in the educational, mental health, and legal systems. Despite challenges associated with family involvement, optimal youth outcomes depend up positive family involvement.

Studies indicate positive family involvement improves treatment compliance, truancy and educational outcome, frequency of suicide attempts, aggression, parenting skills, social development, eating disorders, depression, and anxiety.[45,46] Family involvement typically entails a 3-step process. The first step is to engage families in care. Universal strategies include the creation of an open and welcoming environment. The treatment provider's goal is to improve family input, define what is available to the family, establish protocols for family involvement, and encourage social activities. In the second step, family treatment strategies are more selective. Clinicians must determine specific needs of the family that improve family compliance and provide assistance with resolving family needs. The third step addresses the unique needs of the family and their child. Treatments at this stage are individualized and intensive.[46]

Throughout each step, the clinician must empower the family to speak and be heard, respect the family's perspective, create a collaborative environment, address family needs, address family barriers to care, build off the family's strengths, create opportunities for family involvement, and improve family decision-making.

Immigration and Family Separation

A unique population of youth currently in detention facilities are those who seek asylum or who immigrated to the United States. Asylum seekers and migrants have increased vulnerability for worsened mental health outcomes, thought to be related to premigration experiences of persecution as well as traumas occurring in home countries.[47,40] The postmigration process of seeking asylum may in itself be considered a risk factor, given the trauma associated with interviews or immigration hearings[49] as well as prolonged detention and asylum proceedings.[50]

New US immigration policies have further complicated the process of seeking asylum. In April 2018, under the administration of President Trump, the United States introduced a "zero-tolerance" strategy at the US-Mexico border.[51] Under this policy, all adults entering the United States illegally, even those seeking asylum, were detained and prosecuted. As children cannot be held in federal jails under US law, they were separated from their families and placed in Department of Health and Human Services detention facilities. Estimates report that 2300 children were removed from their parents in 2018.[51] As of December 2020, 628 children remain separated from their families.[52] Among those youth who were reunified with their caregivers, symptoms of social withdrawal, disorientation, and distress were described; in some cases, children were not able to recognize their parents.

The AAP,[53] the American College of Physicians (ACP), and the APA[54] have released statements opposing the separation of children and families due to the risks of considerable harm.[55,56] Before the institution of the "zero-tolerance" strategy, a 2017 report by the AAP reported basic standards of care for children were not being met in detention centers.[53]

Studies on the effects of detention and separation in children are limited. A 2018 systematic review by von Werthern and colleagues found that all detained children met criteria for at least one psychiatric disorder, with affective disorders being most prevalent, including depression, anxiety, and PTSD. Children and their families also reported difficulties with sleep and appetite.[50] Younger children may display developmental difficulties, including delays or regressive behaviors. Existing literature suggests that children who are detained display higher rates of emotional and interpersonal problems as rated by their mothers[55] when compared with scoring guidelines. Male children had higher rates of abnormal peer problems, and younger children had higher rates of abnormal conduct, hyperactivity, and overall difficulty when compared with older children.[49] The length of separation was not found to be significant, implying that any period of separation may be sufficient to cause harm.[55,56] When comparing detained children with asylum seekers in the community, detained children were found to have higher rates of conduct disorder, emotional problems, and hyperactivity.[57] These difficulties persist despite reunification.[58]

Studies to inform best practices in the care of immigrant youth and families postreunification are sparse and primarily focus on children and adolescents who immigrated separately from their parents. Treatment paradigms are focused on trauma-informed care and encourage collaborative models, with participation from health care providers, educators, and community supports.[59] There is no literature available on the long-term treatment of children who were detained and separated from their parents at the time of writing.

SUMMARY

One of the best clinical experiences a psychiatrist can have is working with extremely high-risk youth to help them find safer and better developmental pathways. Few settings can offer such an opportunity to leverage clinical skills to improve the lives and futures of children and adolescents as are afforded to those professionals lucky enough to work in juvenile justice settings. The work is challenging. The work is not without risk. But the work can be a powerful tool to help our patients and our communities.

CLINICS CARE POINTS

- Incarceration, in and of itself, can exacerbate underlying psychiatric illness and create substantial psychosocial risk factors; it should not be undertaken capriciously but only with specific indications and in accordance with prevailing law.

- Psychiatric illnesses, trauma, psychosocial stressors, and social determinants of health are common in justice involved youth and compassionate, evidence-based management is essential to address clinical needs and risk for recidivism.

- Juvenile justice systems disproportionately impact BIPOC youth; clinicians should be sensitive to the potential impact of systemic bias and racism in the experiences of their patients.
- Seclusion, solitary confinement, and unnecessary separation from families can be especially traumatic in juvenile justice and immigration settings.

DISCLOSURE

The authors have nothing to disclose.

REFERENCES

1. US Department of Justice. Office of justice programs. Office of juvenile justice and delinquency prevention. 2015. Available at: http://www.ojjdp.gov/ojstatbb/%20glossary.html. Accessed September 30, 2015.
2. Omboto J, Ondiek G, Odera O, et al. Factors influencing youth crime and juvenile delinquency. Int J Res Social Sci 2013;1(2):18–21.
3. Underwood L, Washington A. Mental illness and juvenile offenders. Int J Environ Res Public Health 2016;13(2):228.
4. Wasserman G, McReynolds L, Lucas D, et al. The voice DISC-IV with incarcerated male youths: prevalence of disorder. J Am Acad Child Adolesc Psychiatry 2002;41:314–21.
5. Fazel S, Doll H. Mental disorders among adolescents in juvenile detention and correctional facilities: a systemic review and metaregression analysis of 25 surveys. J Am Acad Child Adolesc Psychiatry 2008;47(9):1010–9.
6. National Center for Mental Health and Juvenile Justice at Policy Research Associates, Inc, Technical Assistance Collaborative Strengthening Our Future: Key Elements to Developing a Trauma-Informed Juvenile Justice Diversion Program for Youth with Behavioral Health Conditions. 2016. Available at: https://ncyoj.policyresearchinc.org/img/resources/2016-Publication-Strengthening-Our-Future-089881.pdf.
7. Gendraue P, Goggin C. Principles of effective correctional programming. Forum Corrections Res 1996;3:1–6.
8. Gendraue P. The principles of effective intervention with offenders. In: Harland A, editor. Choosing correctional options that work. Thousand oaks (CA): Sage Publications; 1996. p. 38–41.
9. Mental Health America Position Statement 51: Children With Emotional Disorders In The Juvenile Justice System. Mental Health America. Available at: https://www.mhanational.org/issues/position-statement-51-children-emotional-disorders-juvenile-justice-system. Accessed October 14, 2021.
10. Developmental Services Group Intersection between Mental Health and the Juvenile Justice System. Washington, D.C.: Office of Juvenile Justice and Delinquency Prevention; 2017. Available at: https://www.ojjdp.gov/mpg/litreviews/Intersection-Mental-Health-Juvenile-Justice.pdf.
11. Skowyra K., Cocozza JJ. A blueprint for change: Improving the system response to youth with mental health needs involved with the juvenile justice system. National Center for Mental Health and Juvenile Justice; 2006.
12. National Mental Health Association Mental Health Treatment for Youth in the Juvenile Justice System: A Compendium of Promising Practices. Arlington, VA: National Mental health Association; 2004.

13. Abram KM, Teplin LA, Charles DR, et al. Posttraumatic Stress Disorder and trauma in youth in juvenile detention. Arch Gen Psychiatry 2004;61(4):403–10.

14. Ford JD, Grasso DJ, Hawke J, et al. Poly-victimization among juvenile justice involved youths. Child Abuse Negl 2013;37(10):788–800.

15. Saar MS, Epstein R, Rosenthal L, et al. The sexual abuse to prison pipeline: the girls' story. Washington, DC: human rights project for girls, center on poverty and inequality at georgetown law, and Ms. Foundation for Women. 2015. Available at: http://rights4girls.org/wp-content/uploads/r4g/2015/02/2015_C0P_ sexual-abuse_layout_web-1.pdf. Accessed July 19, 2015.

16. Ford J D, Chapman J F, Hawke J, et al. Trauma among youth in the juvenile justice system: Critical issues and new directions. Delmar, NY: National Center for Mental Health and Juvenile Justice; 2007.

17. Perry BD, Pollard RA, Blakley TL, et al. Childhood trauma, the neurobiology of adaptation, and "use-dependent" development of the brain: how "states" become "traits"? Infant Ment Health J 1995;16(4):271–91.

18. Sherman LW, Gottfredson D, MacKenzie D, et al. Preventing crime: what works, what doesn't, what's promising? Washington, DC: Office of Justice Programs; 1997.

19. Harris M, Fallot RD. Envisioning a trauma-informed service system: a vital paradigm shift. New Dir Ment Health Serv 2001;2001(89):3–22.

20. Jewel J, Elliff S. An investigation of the effectiveness of the Relaxation Skills Violence Prevention (RSVP) program with juvenile detainees. Crim Justice Behav 2013;40(2):203–13.

21. Fallot RD, Harris M. A trauma-informed approach to screening and assessment. New Dir Ment Health Serv 2001;89:23–31.

22. Abram KM, Choe JY, Washburn JJ, et al. Suicidal ideation and behaviors among youths in juvenile detention. J Am Acad Child Adolesc Psychiatry 2008;47(3):291–300.

23. Gerson R, Malas N, Feuer V, et al. Best practices for evaluation and treatment of agitated children and adolescents (BETA) in the emergency department: consensus statement of the American Association for Emergency Psychiatry. Western Journal of Emergency Medicine: Integrating Emergency Care with Population Health 2019;20(2):409–18.

24. Richmond JS, Berlin JS, Fishkind AB, et al. Verbal de-escalation of the agitated patient: consensus statement of the American association for emergency Psychiatry project BETA de-escalation Workgroup. West J Emerg Med 2012;13(1):17–25.

25. Drake RE, Bond GR. Psychiatric crisis care and the more is less paradox. Community Ment Health J 2021. https://doi.org/10.1007/s10597-021-00829-2.

26. Rafla-Yuan E, Chhabra DK, Mensah MO. Decoupling crisis response from policing — a step toward equitable psychiatric emergency services. New Engl J Med 2021;384(18):1769–73.

27. Zealberg JJ, Christie SD, Puckett JA, et al. A Mobile crisis program: collaboration between emergency psychiatric services and police. PS 1992;43(6):612–5.

28. Furness T, Maguire T, Brown S, et al. Perceptions of procedural justice and coercion during community-based mental health crisis: a comparison study among stand-alone police response and Co-responding police and mental health clinician response. Policing 2017;11(4):400–9.

29. American Psychiatric Association. Diagnostic and statistical manual of mental disorders: DSM-5. Washington, DC: American Psychiatric Association; 2013. p. 461.

30. Larson K. Best practices for serving court involved youth with learning, attention, and behavioral disabilities. Department of Juvenile Justice, 2002. Available at: http://cecp.air.org/juvenilejustice/docs/promising%20and%Preferred%20Procedures.Pdf Accessed September 30, 2015.
31. McCord J, Tremblay R. Preventing antisocial behavior: interventions from birth through adolescence. New York: Guilford Press; 1992.
32. Kazdin A. Conduct disorders in childhood and adolescence. Thousand Oaks (CA): Sage Publications; 1995.
33. Findling R, Zhou, George P, et al. Diagnostic trends and prescription patterns in disruptive mood dysregulation disorder and bipolar disorder. J Am Acad Child Adolesc Psychiatry 2021.
34. Baglivio MT, Wolff KT, Piquero AR, et al. Racial/ethnic disproportionality in psychiatric diagnoses and treatment in a sample of serious juvenile offenders. J Youth Adolescence 2017;46(7):1424–51.
35. English A, Bass L, Boyle AD, et al. State minor consent laws: a summary. 3rd edition. Center for Adolescent Health Law; 2010. Available at: http://www.cahl.org/state-minor-consent-laws-a-summary-third-edition/.
36. Standards for health services in juvenile detention and confinement facilities. Chicago: National Commission on Correctional Health Care; 2011.
37. Juvenile Justice Reform Committee. Solitary confinement of juvenile of fenders36. Washington, DC: American Academy of Child and Adolescent Psychiatry; 2012.
38. Council of Juvenile Correctional Administrators toolkit: reducing the use of isolation. Braintree (MA): Council of Juvenile Correctional Administrators; 2015. Available at: http://cjca.net. Accessed July 28, 2015.
39. Gagnon JC. The solitary confinement of incarcerated American youth during COVID-19. Psychiatry Res 2020.
40. Trent Maria, Danielle Dooley G, Douge Jacqueline. The impact of racism on child and adolescent mental health. Section on adolescent health, council on community pediatrics, committee on adolescence. Pediatrics 2019;144(2).
41. Ogle Meghan, Turanovic Stephen. The role of race and ethnicity in determini.ng solitary confinements in juvenile detention facilities. College of Criminal Justice. Florida State University; 2019.
42. Marrett Sonja. Beyond rehabilitation: constitutional violations associated with the isolation and discrimination of transgender youth in the juvenile justice system. BCL Rev 2017;58:351.
43. Sedlak AJ, McPherson KS. Youth's needs and services". OJJDP Juv Justice Bull 2010.
44. Braverman PK, Adelman WP. Health care for youth in the juvenile justice system. Pediatrics 2011;128(6):12–9, 1235.
45. Tompson MC, Sugar CA, Langer DA, et al. A Randomized Clinical Trial Comparing Family-Focused Treatment and Individual Supportive Therapy for Depression in Childhood and Early Adolescence. Journal of the American Academy of Child & Adolescent Psychiatry 2017;56(6):515–23.
46. Gopalan G, Goldstein L, Klingenstein K, et al. Engaging Families into Child Mental Health Treatment: Updates and Special Considerations. J Can Acad Child Adolesc Psychiatry 2010;19:182–96.
47. Menjívar C, Perreira KM. Undocumented and unaccompanied: children of migration in the European union and the United States. J Ethnic Migration Stud 2019; 45(2):197–217. https://doi.org/10.1080/1369183X.2017.1404255. Available at:.
48. Priebe S., Giacco D., El-Nagib R. Public health aspects of mental health among migrants and refugees: a review of the evidence on mental health care for

refugees, asylum seekers, and irregular migrants in the WHO European Region (Health Evidence Network Synthesis Report 47). Copenhagen: WHO Regional Office for Europe; 2016.

49. Mares S, Jureidini J. Psychiatric assessment of children and families in immigration detention–clinical, administrative and ethical issues. Aust New Zealand J Public Health 2004;28(6):520–6.

50. Von Werthern M, Robjant K, Chui Z, et al. The impact of immigration detention on mental health: a systematic review. BMC psychiatry 2018;18(1):1–19.

51. Wood LC. Impact of punitive immigration policies, parent-child separation and child detention on the mental health and development of children. BMJ paediatrics open 2018;2(1).

52. Edyburn KL, Meek S. Seeking safety and humanity in the harshest immigration climate in a generation: a review of the literature on the effects of separation and detention on migrant and asylum-seeking children and families in the United States during the Trump administration. Social Policy Rep 2021;34(1):1–46.

53. Linton JM, Griffin M, Shapiro AJ. Detention of immigrant children. Pediatrics 2017; 139(5).

54. Chicco J, Esparza P, Lykes MB, et al. Policy statement on the incarceration of undocumented migrant families: Society for community research and action Division 27 of the American psychological association. Am J Community Psychol 2016.

55. MacLean SA, Agyeman PO, Walther J, et al. Mental health of children held at a United States immigration detention center. Social Sci Med 2019;230:303–8. https://doi.org/10.1016/j.socscimed.2019.04.013. Avaialble at:.

56. MacLean SA, Agyeman PO, Walther J, et al. Characterization of the mental health of immigrant children separated from their mothers at the US–Mexico border. Psychiatry Res 2020;286:112555.

57. Zwi K, Mares S, Nathanson D, et al. The impact of detention on the social–emotional wellbeing of children seeking asylum: a comparison with community-based children. Eur Child Adolesc Psychiatry 2017;27(4):411–22.

58. Lu Y, He Q, Brooks-Gunn J. Diverse experience of immigrant children: how do separation and reunification shape their development? Child Development 2020;91(1):e146–63.

59. Delgado JR, Diaz LD, LaHuffman-Jackson R, et al. Community-based trauma-informed care following immigrant family reunification: a Narrative review. Acad Pediatr 2021;21(4):600–4.

Social and Relational Health Risks and Common Mental Health Problems Among US Children

The Mitigating Role of Family Resilience and Connection to Promote Positive Socioemotional and School-Related Outcomes

Christina D. Bethell, PhD, MBA, MPH[a],*, Andrew S. Garner, MD, PhD[b],
Narangerel Gombojav, MD, PhD[a], Courtney Blackwell, PhD[c],
Laurence Heller, PhD[d], Tamar Mendelson, PhD[a]

KEYWORDS

- Food insecurity • Economic hardship • Neighborhood violence
- Racial discrimination • Relational health • Parent mental health • Parental stress
- Family resilience

Abbreviations	
NSCH	National Survey of Children's Health
MEB	Mental, emotional, and/or behavioral health problems
SHR	Social health risks
RHR	Relational health risks
ACE	Adverse childhood experience
SR	Self-regulation
FRI	Family Resilience Index
PCC	Parent-child connection
CSHCN	Children With Special Health Care Needs
CTC	Communities that Care
PROSPER	Promoting School-University Partnerships to Enhance Resilience
aOR	Adjusted odds ratio

[a] Department of Population, Family and Reproductive Health, Johns Hopkins Bloomberg School of Public Health, Baltimore, MD, USA; [h] Partners in Pediatrics and Case Western Reserve University School of Medicine, Cleveland, OH, USA; [c] Department of Medical Social Sciences, Northwestern University Feinberg School of Medicine, Chicago, IL, USA; [d] NeuroAffective Relational Model Training Institute, Inc, Littleton, CO, USA
* Corresponding author. 615 North Wolfe Street, Room E4152, Baltimore, MD 21205.
E-mail address: cbethell@jhu.edu

Child Adolesc Psychiatric Clin N Am 31 (2022) 45–70
https://doi.org/10.1016/j.chc.2021.08.001
1056-4993/22/© 2021 Elsevier Inc. All rights reserved.

childpsych.theclinics.com

KEY POINTS

- The prevalence of common mental, emotional, and behavioral conditions (MEB) among US children ages 3 to 17 years is 21.8% and varies 4-fold according to the number of relational health risks (RHR) and/or social health risks (SHR) they experience (15.1%–60.4%).
- Nearly 70% (67.6%) of US children aged 3 to 17 years with MEB experience significant RHR (multiple adverse childhood experiences, poor or fair parent/caregiver mental health, high parental stress) and/or SHR (serious economic hardship, food insufficiency, neighborhood violence, racial discrimination) versus 49.3% for children without MEB.
- Children with MEB were nearly half as likely as those without MEB to routinely demonstrate self-regulation (SR; 38.1% vs 73.9%), yet the prevalence of SR for children with MEB varied widely based on their RHR and SHR status (28.3%–50.4%).
- Across all levels of SHR and/or RHR, children with MEB who experienced greater family resilience and parent-child connection were significantly more likely to consistently demonstrate good SR. In turn, this was associated with improved school-related outcomes.
- Child health professionals need to adopt evidence-based preventive, diagnostic, treatment, and counseling approaches that address the mental health impact of children's social and RHR, address the trauma associated with these risks, and build child SR, family resilience skills, and strong parent-child connections. Collaborative, community-based, public health strategies that engage youth, families, as well as health, education, social, and other public services agencies also hold promise.

INTRODUCTION

The increase in child and adolescent mental health problems, suicides, and suicide attempts that have occurred through the coronavirus pandemic[1–4] have confirmed our best science. Positive and adverse social and relational experiences have concrete biologic impacts that shape child development, social and emotional skills, mental health, and overall well-being.[5–8] Socially, children must have basic needs met, like food,[9,10] safe housing,[11] and neighborhoods free from violence[12] and racism.[13] Relationally, healthy development requires the presence of safe, stable, and nurturing relationships across all contexts where children learn, play, and grow.[6,7,14] Efforts to promote mental health and treat mental health problems in children must address their social and community context. Ultimately approaches are needed to repair compromised relationships or establish new ties to caring adults, as well as improve children's social and emotional skills, so they are able to develop and maintain positive relationships throughout life.[5–7,14]

Although Americans value the mental health of children,[15] high rates of diagnosed mental health problems and diminished social and emotional well-being among US children persist along with school and social problems, all of which have long-term impacts on lifelong well-being.[5] At the same time, implementation of evidence-based approaches to prevent or mitigate risks to children's mental health and promote their healthy social and emotional development lags.[5–7,14] A recent synthesis of a series of National Academy of Sciences (NAS) expert reports documents widespread consensus on the urgent need for the United States to prioritize policies that promote the mental health of its children.[16] Common across these reports is a call for integrated and upstream strategies to address the constellation of child-, family-, and community-level risks rather than focusing on single risk factors. Common recommendations include: (1) collaborative efforts across health, education, and social services sectors; (2) team-based approaches to prevent and mitigate risks by proactively promoting child-, family-, and community-level protective factors; (3) training, payment, and performance measurement strategies focused on healthy child development and positive health; and (4) integrated systems of care that address the health and well-being of the whole child and whole family.[16]

There is growing agreement that child primary care, mental health services, and other child-serving community-based services must consider and address children's social and relational health risks (RHR).[5–8,17,18] This includes approaches that address modifiable community-level social health risks (SHR; eg, poverty,[19] food insecurity,[11] exposure to community violence,[12] or racism[13]) and family-level RHR (eg, adverse childhood experiences [ACEs][6,20,21] or caregivers who lack support or are not coping well) that threaten children's healthy physical, mental, social, and relational development and well-being.[22,23] Few studies have evaluated the extent to which community-level SHR versus family-level RHR are differentially associated with children's mental health or are present among children with mental health problems, especially on a population basis for all US children. Such information is critical to inform and improve the methods that health care organizations and other child and youth-serving agencies use to assess and pursue opportunities to promote positive child mental health and reduce risks to the mental health of children.

Similarly, although many studies focus on single SHR or RHR, population-based studies that examine the complexity (eg, experiencing both SHR and RHR) and cumulative impact of a range of evidence-based social and relational risks to children's mental health are few. Such studies are needed to inform policy and practice and are especially relevant given strong evidence pointing to the impact of cumulative (vs single) risks and the common toxic stress-related neurobiological and developmental pathways through which SHR and RHR can impact child mental health, regardless of the specific risk involved.[6,7,14]

National, state, and local policymakers and child health services programs, family and community leaders, and professionals need to better understand and mitigate the impact of SHR and RHR on children's mental health and promote resilience. In this, data demonstrating how, at a population level these types of risks co-occur, interact, and are associated with healthy child development and school and social outcomes is essential. It is especially important to foster understanding about how the toxic stress and trauma associated with RHR and SHR may be impacting the development of essential positive social and emotional skills, such as self-regulation (SR) of emotions and behavior, and, in turn, the academic and social functioning of US children.[6,8,21,24–30] Such an understanding is key to the translation of existing evidence-based approaches shown to promote positive social and emotional skills and resilience, even among children experiencing toxic stress and trauma and mental, emotional, and behavioral problem (MEB) symptoms related to current or past SHR and RHR.[6,27,31–35] In turn, this can reduce behaviors resulting in diminished academic and social functioning, like reduced school engagement and attendance and/or bullying victimization and/or perpetration.[6,8,21,26,29,30,36–38]

Further elucidating at a population level, the mitigatable protective factors that can reduce negative impacts of SHR and RHR is also important to inform effective child mental health promotion, prevention, and treatment policies and practices. In particular, a positive parent-child bond has been identified as perhaps the most critical factor for healthy child development and positive mental health and flourishing, with potential to strongly buffer against substantial SHR and RHR exposure.[6,7,14,33–35,39–45] Family resilience, which has been conceptualized as the capacity of the family system to withstand stressors and maintain positive functioning, has also been shown in emerging research to offer another source of protection against the negative effects of SHR and/or RHR on children's SR and mental health.[22,40,43,46,47]

In this study, we leveraged nationally representative data on US children to advance population-based knowledge and inform efforts to prevent and optimize positive mental health for all US children. Specifically, we (1) estimated the prevalence of evidence-based SHR and RHR among US children with and without MEB; (2) examined variations in the prevalence of MEB among US children based on their SHR and RHR; (3) explored associations between the SHR and RHR experienced by children with MEB and their SR skills, engagement and attendance in school and school-based bullying victimization and/or perpetration; and (4) examined whether greater family resilience and parent-child connection (PCC) is associated with stronger SR skills among children with MEB and SHR and/or RHR and, in turn, improved school engagement and attendance and reduced bullying victimization and/or perpetration.

METHODS
Data and Population

We used data from a combined 2016 to 2019 National Survey of Children's Health (NSCH; n = 131,774) data set we created for this study.[48,49] The NSCH is an annual survey led by the US Health Resources and Services Administration's (HRSA) Maternal and Child Health Bureau (MCHB) in collaboration with the US Bureau of the Census.[48] The NSCH relies on address-based sampling and is self-administered by the caregiver (parent or guardian) of a randomly selected child (age 0–17 years) in sampled households. Missing value rates were less than 3% for any individual item used in the study, which is well under the suggested 5% to 10%.[50] This study evaluated data for children ages 3 to 17 years. All data were weighted and adjusted for the complex sampling design of the NSCH to produce estimates representative of all children nationally and across states. See Appendix A1 for further details.[51]

KEY MEASURES

Below is a summary of variables used in this study. See Ref. 49 and Appendix A2 for further detail on the scoring of each measure.[51]

Mental, Emotional, and Behavioral Conditions

Children were identified as having MEB if (1) their caregiver/parent indicated that their child currently experienced any type of ongoing MEB that requires treatment or counseling as reported using the Children with Special Health Care Needs (CSHCN) Screener[52]; and/or (2) their caregiver reported that the child currently has one or more of 10 mental health conditions that a doctor told them their child had, including depression, anxiety, conduct/behavior disorder, attention-deficit/hyperactivity disorder (ADHD), a learning disability, autism, developmental delay, intellectual disability, Tourette syndrome, or speech disorder.[49]

Social Health Risks and Relational Health Risks Variables

We optimized data available in the NSCH to specify robust and parsimonious SHR and RHR indices each made up of risks documented to be associated with child mental health. We built on Sameroff and colleague's approach, whereby risk measures were selected based on: (1) prominent models and measures with significant literature basis on the risk's impact on child mental health and development; (2) high reliability of individual risk measures; and (3) nonredundant information provided by individual measures assessed based on across-measure correlation findings.[53,54] We also sought to identify measures aligned with prominent social determinants of health (SDOH) assessments used in the field, such as the Accountable Health Communities (AHC) Health-Related Social Needs (HRSN) Screening Tool and the Safe Environment for Every Kid (SEEK) screener.[55,56] See Appendix A4 for a cross-walk between the SHR and RHR specified for this study and the AHC-HRSN and other SDOH screening instruments.[51]

We used dichotomous high/low cutoff scores for each measure, with specific criteria based on values known to be predictive of child mental health outcomes or clinical/diagnostic criteria.[5,8,49,57] When setting cutoffs, we took a conservative approach that errs on the side of positive predictive value over negative predictive value such that if a child was positively identified on any measure, there would be unarguable evidence that the child was at risk (eg, children met cutoff criteria if *caregivers* reported "poor or fair" overall mental health status even though "good" reports often suggest children are at increased risk compared to those with "very good" and "excellent" ratings[58,59]). Below, we provide an overview of individual measures constructed using the NSCH that were included in the SHR and RHR composite variables.

The *SHR* index includes 4 measures prior research documents are associated with child mental health. These SHR measures identify children whose caregivers reported that they: (1) sometimes or often could not afford enough food to eat[9,10]; (2) experienced serious economic hardship and somewhat often or very often found it hard to cover the costs of basics needs, including housing[19]; (3) lived in an unsafe neighborhood or where the child was a victim of or witnessed violence[12]; and (4) witnessed their child being treated or judged unfairly because of his or her race or ethnic group.[13] Pearson's correlations among the 4 SHR measures were evaluated to assess information redundancy, which we sought to minimize. Correlation ranged from 0.06 to 0.37 and each was low using standard intervals established in the literature to evaluate the strength of correlations ($r = 0$, *no correlation;* $r =$ below ± 0.10, *low*; $r = \pm 0.30$, *moderate*; $r \geq \pm 0.50$, *large*; $r = 1$, *perfect correlation*) with one moderate correlation (0.37 correlation between serious economic hardship and food insecurity).[60]

The RHR index includes 4 measures that prior research documents are associated with children's social and emotional skills and mental health. These measures identify children who: (1) ever experienced 2 or more of 6 household level ACEs using the validated NSCH_ACEs indicator (serious parental mental illness, household substance, drug or alcohol abuse, witnessed domestic violence, parental death, divorce/separation, or incarceration)[6,20,21,61]; (2) had 1 or 2 caregivers with fair/poor mental health[5,8,10,62–64]; (3) had a caregiver report frequent aggravation with their child[23]; and (4) had a caregiver who lacked emotional support or was not coping well.[22] Pearson's correlations among the 4 RHR measures were evaluated to assess information redundancy. Correlation ranged from 0.04 to 0.18 and each was low using standard intervals established in the literature to evaluate the strength of correlations.[60] Correlations across all 8 SHR and RHR index measurement criteria ranged from 0.03 to 0.37.

RHR and SHR scoring: First, we created SHR and RHR count variables indicating whether a child experienced 0, 1, or 2 to 4 of the SHR and RHR evaluated. We then created a mutually exclusive combinations composite variable indicating whether children experienced any number of (1) both SHR and RHR; (2) SHR only; (3) RHR only; or (4) neither RHR and SHR. See Appendix A2 for details on each SHR and RHR criteria and Appendix A3 for correlations across SHR and RHR individual measures.[51]

CHILD HEALTH OUTCOMES AND FAMILY PROTECTIVE FACTORS

Four child health outcomes associated with child exposure to SHR and RHR and their mental health were evaluated: SR skills, engagement in school, school attendance, and bullying victimization and/or perpetration. Two family protective factors variables included the Family Resilience Index (FRI) and an indicator of PCC. Specification of each of these variables is summarized below.

Child Self-regulation

The child SR measure available in the NSCH provides an overall evaluation of whether children demonstrate the ability to "bounce back quickly when things to not go their way" (age 3–5 years) or "stay calm and in control when faced with a challenge" (age 6–17 years). These measures were developed and validated for use in the NSCH as part of a larger child flourishing index[40,65] that assesses a child's capacity for regulating stimulus-driven emotion and physiologic stress response systems and the capacity for avoiding inappropriate or aggressive actions. This indicator of a child's SR skills represents an important subconstruct within broader definitions of child SR and is strongly associated with the ability of children to have positive interactions with others and the ability to carry out self-directed learning.[31,32] Children were identified as "consistently demonstrating self-regulation skills" if their caregivers reported "definitely true" (2016–2017 NSCH) or "usually/always" to the NSCH SR items.

Engagement in School

School-age children ages 6 to 17 years met criteria for school engagement if their caregivers reported that their child "cares about doing well in school" and "does all required homework."

Missed School

Children ages 6 to 17 years were identified as missing more than 2 or more weeks of school in the past years if they were enrolled in school and their caregiver reported that they missed 11 or more school days because of an illness or injury during the past 12 months.

Bullying Victimization and/or Perpetration

This measure was constructed by combining caregiver/parent responses to 2 questions assessing whether in the past 12 months their child was (1) bullied, picked on, or excluded other children and/or (2) bullied, picked on, or excluded by other children. These questions were asked for children ages 6 to 17 years and were combined because of their co-occurring nature at the child level.

Parent-Child Connection

Whether children experience strong "PCC" was assessed for children ages 6 to 17 years based on caregiver responses to the question "How well can you and this child share ideas or talk about things that really matter?"

Family Resilience Index

Whether children live in a family that consistently practices resilience skills was assessed using the validated, 4-item NSCH FRI,[40] which asks caregivers how often, when their family faces problems, they talk together about what to do, work together to solve their problem, know they have strengths to draw on and stay hopeful in difficult times.

Other Child Characteristics

Other measures used in this study included child age (3–5, 6–11, and 12–17 years); sex (male = 1, female = 0); race and ethnicity (Hispanic, Non-Hispanic Black, Non-Hispanic White, and Other/Multiracial); household poverty level (calculated as a percentage of the federal poverty level; 0%–99%, 100%–199%, 200%–399%, and $\geq$ 400%); and type of health insurance (public, uninsured, and private).

ANALYTICAL PROCEDURES
Prevalence of Social Health Risks and Relational Health Risks and Variations in Mental, Emotional, and/Or Behavioral Health Problems Among all US Children by Their Social Health Risks and Relational Health Risks (Study Aim 1 and 2)

SHR and RHR prevalence rates were constructed and evaluated for all children ages 3 to 17 years with and without MEB, by specific MEB conditions (eg, depression, anxiety, conduct disorder, ADHD) and for all other key study variables. MEB prevalence rates were calculated for all US children ages 3 to 17 years and separately for children in each of the 4 SHR and RHR mutually exclusive combination categories as well as their SHR and RHR measure count score and for each of the 8 individual SHR and RHR measures. MEB prevalence was also calculated by all study outcomes and protective factors and child characteristics described earlier. Chi-square tests were used to assess the significance of all observed differences. Multivariable logistic regression analyses were used to calculate adjusted odds ratios (aORs) to evaluate the significance and magnitude of observed associations and variations after adjusting for children's age, sex, race/ethnicity, household poverty level, and insurance status/type.

Evaluating Associations Between Child's Self-regulation Skills and Their School Engagement, Missed School and Bullying/Bullied Outcomes by Social Health Risks and Relational Health Risks (Study Aim 3)

Multivariable logistic regression analyses were used to evaluate associations between each of the 3 school-related study outcomes (engagement in school, missed school, bullying victimization and/or perpetration) and children's (1) SR and (2) SHR and RHR status. Stratified logistic regression models were used to assess differences in associations between school-related outcomes and children's SR status overall and separately for mutually exclusive SHR and RHR subgroup (both SHR/RHR, SHR only, RHR only, neither).

Estimating Associations Between Children's Self-regulation and Their Family Resilience and Parent-Child Connection Status Across Social Health Risks and Relational Health Risks Subgroups (Study Aim 4)

We conducted a series of multivariate logistic regression analyses to evaluate associations between children's SR status and their family resilience and PCC status. Analyses were conducted for all children with MEB and separately for children with MEB based on their SHR and RHR status.

All regression analyses controlled for children's sex, age, race/ethnicity, household poverty level, and insurance status/type. Results are presented as aORs with 95% confidence intervals (95% CI). All analyses were conducted using SPSS version 25 (IBM).

RESULTS
Prevalence of Social Health Risks and Relational Health Risks Among US Children with Mental, Emotional, and/or Behavioral Health Problems (Study Aim 1)

Nearly 70% (67.6%) of US children ages 3 to 17 years with MEB experienced RHR and/or SHR versus 49.3% for children without MEB. RHR were more common than

SHR among children with MEB (56% vs 42.5%, P<.001). Serious economic hardship was the most prevalent SHR (31.7%) and having 2 or more household level ACEs was the most prevalent RHR (28.5%) (**Table 1**).

Variations in Mental, Emotional, and/or Behavioral Health Problems Prevalence by the Social Health Risks and Relational Health Risks Status of Children (Study Aim 2)

The prevalence of MEB among US children ages 3 to 17 years was 21.8% and varied 4-fold (15.1%–60.4%, P<.001) across groups of children according to both the type and amount of RHR and SHR they experienced (**Fig. 1**). Children with any or both SHR and RHR were more likely to have MEB compared to children with neither type of risk. Children with 2 to 4 RHR were more likely to have MEB than children with 2 to 4 SHR (50.1% vs 41.6%, P<.001; see **Table 1**). As shown in **Fig. 1**, 60.4% of US children ages 3 to 17 years had MEB if they experienced both 2 to 4 SHR and 2 to 4 RHR, whereas 28.8% of children with 2 to 4 SHR and no RHR had MEB and 42.3% of children had MEB if they had 2 to 4 RHR and no SHR. See **Fig. 1** for more in-depth findings and aORs associated with these comparisons. See Appendix B2 for regression details associated with **Fig. 1**.

The prevalence of specific MEB conditions was higher for children who experienced SHR and/or RHR. This was especially true for depression, conduct disorder, and anxiety. For instance, children had 9.17 greater odds (95% CI, 7.64–11.00) of having depression if they experienced both SHR and RHR than if they experienced neither type of risk. Overall, having any RHR was more strongly associated with most of the specific MEB conditions assessed as compared with having SHR only. See **Table 2** for detailed findings.

Additional findings on the prevalence and characteristics of US children with MEB can be found in **Table 1** (eg, age, sex, race/ethnicity, type of health insurance). Of note, once adjusted for SHR, the prevalence of MEB was slightly, but significantly, lower for non-white and lower-income children across all levels of RHR (see Appendix B2). In addition, publicly insured children were 1.56 times more likely to have MEB than privately insured children (28.6% vs 18.3%, P<.001).

School-Related Outcomes Among Children with Mental, Emotional, and/Or Behavioral Health Problems by Their Self-regulation and Social Health Risks and Relational Health Risks Status (Study Aim 3)

Overall, US children aged 3 to 17 years with MEB were nearly half as likely as those without MEB to consistently demonstrate good SR skills (38.1% vs 73.9%, P<.001; see **Table 1**). Yet, the prevalence of children with MEB who consistently demonstrated SR varied from 28.3% for those with both SHR and RHR to 50.4% for children with neither type of risk (P<.001; aOR, 0.45; 95% CI, 0.38–0.53). See **Tables 3** and **4** for additional findings.

US children ages 6 to 17 years with MEB were nearly 2 times more likely to engage in school if they consistently demonstrated good SR skills (74.7% vs 39.1%; RR, 1.91). Said differently, compared to school-age children with MEB demonstrating SR, those with poorer SR had 77% lower odds of engaging in school (aOR, 0.23; 95% CI, 0.20–0.26). Similarly, children not consistently demonstrating good SR had 1.60 times greater odds (95% CI, 1.29–1.97) of missing 2 or more weeks of schools in the past year (11.1% vs 7.2%, P<.001) and 1.37 times greater odds (95% CI, 1.21–1.54) of bullying victimization and/or perpetration (61.5% vs 53%, P<.001) compared to children with MEB who did demonstrate SR (see **Table 3**).

The prevalence of each of these outcomes also varied according to children's SHR and RHR status. Across the 4 SHR/RHR mutually exclusive groups, school

Table 1
Prevalence and characteristics of US children who have one or more of the common MEB assessed in the National Survey of Children's Health.

Child Characteristics	Prevalence of MEB by Child Characteristics		Among All Children		Prevalence of Child Characteristics by MEB Status			
					Among Children MEB		Children Without MEB	
	n	%	n	%	n	%	N	%
All children, aged 3–17 y	27,433	21.8%	114,476	100	27,433	21.8%	87,043	78.2%
Age, y [a,b]								
3–5	2537	13.1%	20,107	19.4%	2537	11.7%	17,570	21.6%
6–11	9679	22.2%	39,935	40.1%	9679	41.0%	30,256	39.9%
12–17	15,217	25.5%	54,434	40.4%	15,217	47.4%	39,217	38.5%
Sex [a,b]								
Male	16,070	25.5%	59,116	51.1%	16,070	59.9%	43,046	48.7%
Female	11,363	17.9%	55,360	48.9%	11,363	40.1%	43,997	51.3%
Race/ethnicity [a,b]								
Hispanic	3031	19.3%	13,131	25.3%	3031	22.5%	10,100	26.1%
White, Non-Hispanic	19,779	23.6%	79,637	50.5%	19,779	54.7%	59,858	49.4%
Black, Non-Hispanic	1832	23.3%	7224	13.6%	1832	14.6%	5392	13.4%
Other, Non-Hispanic	2791	17.1%	14,484	10.5%	2791	8.2%	11,693	11.1%
Income level (FPL) [a,b]								
0%–99% FPL	3891	26.0%	12,643	20.2%	3891	24.2%	8752	19.1%
100%–199% FPL	4984	23.0%	18,351	21.9%	4984	23.1%	13,367	21.6%
200%–399% FPL	8320	20.6%	35,271	27.3%	8320	25.8%	26,951	27.8%
400% FPL or more	10,238	19.2%	48,211	30.5%	10,238	26.9%	37,973	31.5%
Insurance status and type [a,b]								
Has public insurance	9347	28.6%	26,111	35.2%	9347	46.2%	16,764	32.1%

(continued on next page)

Table 1
(continued)

Child Characteristics	Prevalence of MEB by Child Characteristics		Among All Children		Prevalence of Child Characteristics by MEB Status			
					Among Children MEB		Children Without MEB	
	n	%	n	%	n	%	N	%
Has private insurance only	16,701	18.3%	81,844	58.2%	16,701	48.9%	65,143	60.8%
Is uninsured	983	16.1%	4773	6.7%	983	4.9%	3790	7.1%
SHR and RHR status[a,b]								
Has both SHR and RHR	6916	39.5%	14,960	16.9%	6916	30.8%	8044	13.1%
Has SHR, not RHR	2809	23.1%	10,928	11.0%	2809	11.7%	8119	10.9%
Has RHR, not SHR	7117	21.6%	25,579	25.3%	7117	25.1%	18,462	25.4%
Has neither SHR nor RHR	10,225	15.1%	61,342	46.7%	10,225	32.4%	51,117	50.7%
SHR criteria count[a,b]								
0	17,345	17.4%	86,941	72.0%	17,345	57.5%	69,596	76.0%
1	6351	29.0%	18,681	19.1%	6351	25.4%	12,330	17.3%
2–4	3375	41.6%	7213	8.9%	3375	17.1%	3838	6.7%
Specific SHR criteria								
Food insecurity: Sometimes or often could not afford enough to eat[a,b]	1995	38.4%	4621	6.1%	1995	10.7%	2626	4.8%
Serious economic hardship: Somewhat often/very often hard to cover costs of basic needs, like food, housing[a,b]	7173	34.2%	18,775	20.2%	7173	31.7%	11,602	17.0%
Neighborhood safety/violence: Lived in an unsafe neighborhood or where the child was a victim of or witnessed violence[a,b]	3409	39.5%	7485	8.9%	3409	16.1%	4076	6.8%
Racial discrimination: Child has been treated or judged unfairly because of their race/ethnic group[a,b]	1471	34.4%	3927	4.6%	1471	7.3%	2456	3.8%
RHR criteria count[a,b]								

	N	%	N	%	N	%	N	%
0	13,163	16.7%	72,858	57.8%	13,163	44.3%	59,695	61.5%
1	8862	22.7%	31,280	32.9%	8862	34.2%	22,418	32.5%
2–4	5243	50.1%	9488	9.3%	5243	21.4%	4245	6.0%
Specific RHR criteria								
Multiple ACEs: Exposed to 2 or more household level ACEs[a,b]	7044	41.2%	15,947	15.1%	7044	28.5%	8903	11.3%
Poor/Fair caregiver mental health: 1 or 2 caregivers reported poor or fair mental health[a,b]	3566	42.5%	8090	7.5%	3566	14.7%	4524	5.5%
Parental aggravation: Child's caregiver usually/always felt aggravated with child[a,b]	4671	71.1%	6001	5.4%	4671	17.5%	1330	2.0%
Poor parent coping/support: Child's caregiver is coping not very well or not well at all and or lacks emotional support[a,b]	5724	20.1%	22,490	26.3%	5724	24.3%	16,766	26.9%
SR[a,b]								
Consistently demonstrated good SR (definitely true; always/usually true)	10,295	12.6%	74,351	66.1%	10,295	38.1%	64,056	73.9%
Did not consistently demonstrate good SR (somewhat true or sometimes)	13,518	35.5%	34,520	30.0%	13,518	48.8%	21,002	24.7%
Not true or never	3291	72.2%	4241	4.0%	3291	13.2%	950	1.4%
School engagement, ages 6–17 y[a,b]								
Engaged in school	12,758	16.3%	69,634	75.6%	12,758	51.7%	56,876	83.1%
Did not engage in school	11,883	47.4%	23,721	24.4%	11,883	48.3%	11,838	16.9%
Missed school days, ages 6–17 y[a,b]								
0–10 d in past year	21,984	22.5%	88,746	95.9%	21,984	90.4%	66,762	97.6%
11+ d/2+ wk in past year	2439	56.2%	3968	4.1%	2439	9.6%	1529	2.4%
Bullying victimization and/or perpetration, ages 6–17 y[a,b]								
Yes	14,286	38.3%	34,984	36.5%	14,286	58.4%	20,698	29.6%
No	10,358	15.7%	58,352	63.5%	10,358	41.6%	47,994	70.4%

(continued on next page)

Table 1
(continued)

| Child Characteristics | Prevalence of MEB by Child Characteristics | | Prevalence of Child Characteristics by MEB Status | | | | | |
| | | | Among All Children | | Among Children MEB | | Children Without MEB | |
	n	%	n	%	n	%	N	%
FRI score[a,b]								
Met 0–1 criterion	14,928	26.1%	53,184	42.9%	14,928	51.3%	38,256	40.5%
Met 2–3 criteria	5288	20.6%	22,921	20.4%	5288	19.3%	17,633	20.8%
Met all 4 criteria	6901	17.5%	36,802	36.7%	6901	29.4%	29,901	38.7%
Parent-Child connection, ages 6–17 y: Parents and children share ideas or talk about things that really matter[a,b]								
Very well	12,131	17.5%	61,364	66.9%	12,131	49.0%	49,233	72.6%
Somewhat well	9456	32.4%	27,245	28.6%	9456	38.6%	17,789	25.4%
Not very well or not well at all	2932	65.7%	4099	4.5%	2932	12.4%	1167	2.0%

Data for ages 3–17 years unless otherwise noted.

Abbreviation: FPL, federal poverty level.

[a] Indicates that differences in the prevalence of MEB across child characteristic are statistically significant at the *P* value less than .001 level of significance.

[b] Indicates that differences in the prevalence of child characteristics and SHR and/or RHR between children with or without MEB are statistically significant at the *P* value less than .001 level of significance.

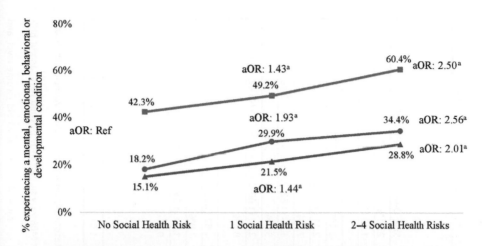

Fig. 1. Prevalence of US children age 3 to 17 years who experienced an MEB, by their SHR and RHR criteria count. Data: 2016 to 2019 National Survey of Children's Health. Notes. All prevalence rates are weighted to represent the US child population ages 3 to 17 years. aORs are adjusted for age, sex, race/ethnicity, income and insurance coverage type. [a]aORs are statistically significant after adjusting for age, sex, race/ethnicity, income and insurance coverage type. See Technical Appendix B1 for detailed stratified regression analysis findings.

engagement ranged from 41.4% to 64.0% (P<.001) and aORs engagement in school was 28% to 53% lower for children with MEB who experienced SHR and/or RHR compared to those with neither type of risk (see Appendix C1). The prevalence of children with MEB who missed 2 or more weeks of school in the past year ranged from 4.4% to 14.8% (P<.001) across SHR/RHR subgroups (aORs ranged from 1.99 to 3.41). The prevalence of bullying victimization and/or perpetration ranged from 49.1% to 70.4% (P<.001) across SHR/RHR subgroups (aORs ranged from 1.33 to 2.68). All aORs were statistically significant for all 3 outcomes (see Appendix C1).

Findings on associations between the SR and school engagement status of children with MEB were consistent when separately evaluated across each mutually exclusive subgroup of children according to their SHR and RHR status (both SHR/RHR, SHR only, RHR only, neither). As shown in **Fig. 2**, across each SHR/RHR subgroup, children with MEB were 3.06 to 3.75 times more likely to engage in school if they had good versus poor SR skills. See **Fig. 2** and Appendix D1 for regression details associated with **Fig. 2**. See Appendix D2 and D3 for regression details and results for the "missed school" and bullying victimization and/or perpetration outcomes. Of note, although both higher SR and exposure to SHR and/or RHR were independently associated with higher prevalence of missed school and bullying victimization and/or perpetration, aORs comparing these outcomes across SHR and RHR subgroups for children with and without stronger SR were significant only for children with RHR only (see **Table 3**).

Self-regulation Among Children with Mental, Emotional, and/or Behavioral Health Problems by Their Family Resilience, Parent-Child Connection and Social Health Risks and Relational Health Risks Status (Study Aim 4)

Children with MEB who experienced greater family resilience and PCC were significantly more likely to consistently demonstrate good SR skills (see **Table 4**). As shown

Table 2
Prevalence and adjusted odds ratios of specific MEB among US children overall and by their SR and SHR and RHR status.

Children's Common MEB Conditions	Prevalence Among all US Children, Ages 3–17 y	Prevalence by child's SR status[a]		Prevalence by child's SHR and RHR status[b,c]			
		Consistently Demonstrated Good SR	Did Not Consistently Demonstrate Good SR	Both SHR and RHR	SHR Only	RHR Only	Neither
Experiences any MEB[c]	21.8%	12.6%	39.8%	39.5%	23.1%	21.6%	15.1%
Adjusted odds ratios		Ref	4.32 (4.04–4.63)	3.63 (3.29–4.00)	1.70 (1.51–1.91)	1.56 (1.44–1.69)	Ref
Specific MEB							
Depression	3.4%	1.5%	7.2%	9.8%	2.4%	3.7%	1.2%
Adjusted odds ratios		Ref	5.12 (4.41–5.94)	9.17 (7.64–11.00)	2.11 (1.67–2.68)	3.29 (2.78–3.88)	Ref
Anxiety	7.8%	3.8%	15.6%	17.0%	7.1%	7.8%	4.6%
Adjusted odds ratios		Ref	4.64 (4.21–5.12)	5.30 (4.69–5.99)	1.88 (1.62–2.18)	1.97 (1.77–2.18)	Ref
Conduct/Behavior disorder	7.0%	1.8%	17.1%	17.8%	5.9%	7.9%	2.8%
Adjusted odds ratios		Ref	9.93 (8.76–11.26)	6.93 (5.87–8.18)	2.03 (1.68–2.46)	2.94 (2.52–3.42)	Ref
Attention-deficit disorder or ADHD	8.7%	3.9%	18.2%	16.5%	8.6%	9.4%	5.7%
Adjusted odds ratios		Ref	5.00 (4.57–5.47)	3.13 (2.75–3.55)	1.57 (1.35–1.84)	1.72 (1.53–1.93)	Ref
Learning disability	6.9%	3.3%	13.9%	14.5%	7.9%	6.9%	3.8%
Adjusted odds ratios		Ref	4.15 (3.70–4.65)	3.27 (2.82–3.79)	1.87 (1.54–2.27)	1.60 (1.39–1.84)	Ref
Child meets criteria for having a special health care need that involves any type of MEB requiring treatment or counseling	9.7%	3.5%	21.8%	22.3%	9.2%	11.0%	4.5%
Adjusted odds ratios		Ref	4.73 (4.23–5.29)	3.87 (3.29–4.55)	1.51 (1.25–1.83)	2.76 (2.41–3.17)	Ref

Data for ages 3–17 years unless otherwise noted.

[a] Indicates that all observed differences in the prevalence of specific MEB conditions by child's SR status are statistically significant at the P value less than .001 level of significance and all adjusted odds ratios are also significant.

[b] Indicates that all differences in the prevalence of specific MEB conditions between children with or without MEB vary significantly by child's SHR and/or RHR status at the P value less than .001 level of significance and all adjusted odds ratios are also significant.

[c] See **Fig. 1** for further details on MEB prevalence by SHR and RHR status. aORs are adjusted for child's age, sex, race-ethnicity, household income level, and insurance status/type.

Table 3

Variations in the prevalence of school-related outcomes among children aged 6–17 years with MEB who do or do not consistently demonstrate good SR[a], for all children and by their social and relational risk status

	Prevalence of Outcomes for all Children Ages 6–17 y with MEB		Prevalence of Outcomes by the SHR and RHR Status (Among Children Ages 6–17 y with MEB)							
			Both SHR and RHR		SHR, Not RHR		RHR, Not SHR		Neither SHR nor RHR	
	%	aOR	%	aOR	%	aOR	%	aOR	%	aOR
Prevalence of children who consistently demonstrated good SR, ages 6–17 y	38.1%	NA	28.3%	NA	38.3%	NA	33.6%	NA	50.4%	NA
Prevalence of children with MEB who engaged in school, 6–17 y										
Consistently demonstrated good SR	74.7%	Ref	66.8%	Ref	75.3%	Ref	74.9%	Ref	79.9%	Ref
Did not consistently demonstrate good SR	39.1%	0.23 (0.20–0.26)	32.4%	0.24 (0.18–0.32)	40.0%	0.24 (0.15–0.37)	36.7%	0.20 (0.15–0.26)	49.3%	0.24 (0.19–0.29)
Prevalence among children with MEB who missed 2 wk or more school days, 6–17 y										
Consistently demonstrated good SR	7.2%	Ref	13.3%	Ref	9.0%	Ref	6.7%	Ref	4.1%	Ref
Did not consistently demonstrate good SR	11.1%	1.60 (1.29–1.97)	15.5%	1.24 (0.86–1.79)	13.4%	1.64 (0.84–3.19)	9.9%	1.71 (1.22–2.39)	4.6%	1.21 (0.85–1.72)
Prevalence of children with MEB who experienced victimization and/or perpetration of bullying, 6–17 y										
Consistently demonstrated good SR	53.0%	Ref	66.8%	Ref	60.6%	Ref	46.9%	Ref	46.7%	Ref
Did not consistently demonstrate good SR	61.5%	1.37 (1.21–1.54)	71.8%	1.27 (0.96–1.67)	55.6%	0.83 (0.57–1.21)	59.6%	1.71 (1.35–2.16)	51.4%	1.16 (0.98–1.37)

[a] SR categorized into 2 groups because of sample size limitations.

Table 4
Prevalence of US children ages 3–17 years with MEB who with good SR, by their family resilience and parent-child connection status

	Prevalence of Children with MEB Who Consistently Demonstrated Good SR		Prevalence of Children with MEB Who Demonstrated Good SR by Their SHR and RHR Status							
			Among Children with MEB Experiencing Both SHR and RHR		Among Children with MEB Experiencing SHR, But Not RHR		Among Children with MEB Experiencing RHR, But Not SHR		Among Children with MEB Experiencing Neither SHR nor RHR	
	%	aOR	%	aOR	%	aOR	%	aOR	%	aOR
All children with MEB	38.1%	N/A	28.3%	0.45 (0.38–0.53)	38.3%	0.66 (0.54–0.81)	33.6%	0.53 (0.46–0.61)	50.4%	Ref
FRI score: (4 items-family talks, problem solves, maintains hope, recognizes strengths)										
0–1	32.2%	Ref	24.7%	Ref	35.3%	Ref	27.2%	Ref	46.0%	Ref
2–3	39.6%	1.44 (1.24–1.67)	28.0%	1.28 (0.90–1.81)	34.1%	1.03 (0.65–1.64)	37.8%	1.83 (1.36–2.44)	52.3%	1.31 (1.07–1.59)
All 4	46.8%	1.99 (1.73–2.28)	38.1%	2.03 (1.47–2.81)	45.3%	1.77 (1.11–2.81)	43.5%	2.23 (1.72–2.90)	54.5%	1.53 (1.27–1.84)
Parent-Child connection, ages 6–17 y: Parent-child share ideas and talk about things that really matter										
Very well	46.5%	5.73 (4.54–7.23)	35.7%	4.75 (3.07–7.35)	44.9%	10.04 (4.52–22.30)	42.8%	6.24 (4.42–8.81)	55.7%	3.44 (2.16–5.49)
Somewhat well	29.5%	2.68 (2.11–3.42)	23.6%	2.49 (1.57–3.94)	28.6%	4.59 (2.00–10.52)	26.5%	2.82 (1.96–4.05)	38.8%	1.70 (1.06–2.74)
Not very well, at all	12.8%	Ref	11.4%	Ref	7.0%	Ref	11.2%	Ref	25.1%	Ref
Detailed findings by specific FRI measures illustrating variations in associations with SR by "All of the time" vs. "Most of the time" responses to FRI items										
Family knows they have strengths to draw on when the family faces problems										
All of the time	44.7%	2.26 (1.85–2.76)	34.7%	1.78 (1.24–2.54)	42.7%	1.56 (0.73–3.31)	40.7%	2.49 (1.88–3.30)	54.1%	2.10 (1.52–2.92)
Most of the time	35.2%	1.46 (1.20–1.78)	25.6%	1.13 (0.80–1.59)	34.4%	0.99 (0.47–2.10)	30.3%	1.53 (1.17–2.00)	47.5%	1.56 (1.12–2.18)
None/some of the time	25.7%	Ref	23.9%	Ref	30.5%	Ref	22.3%	Ref	36.8%	Ref
Family stays hopeful even in difficult times when the family faces problems										
All of the time	43.9%	2.39 (1.87–3.05)	33.4%	1.80 (1.19–2.70)	42.4%	2.39 (1.21–4.72)	40.7%	2.57 (1.80–3.66)	54.0%	1.89 (1.17–3.06)
Most of the time	34.2%	1.40 (1.10–1.77)	24.7%	1.05 (0.72–1.53)	34.9%	1.42 (0.71–2.82)	28.5%	1.29 (0.91–1.83)	46.7%	1.31 (0.81–2.12)
None/some of the time	26.0%	Ref	25.1%	Ref	25.5%	Ref	22.9%	Ref	40.8%	Ref

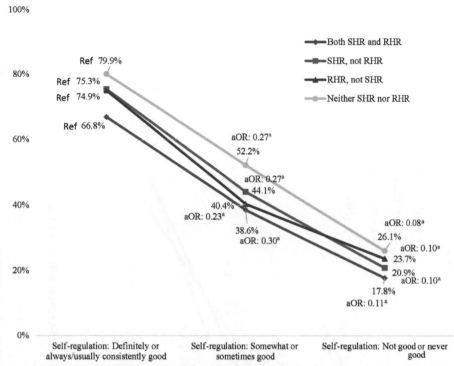

Fig. 2. Prevalence of US children age 6 to 17 years with MEB who were engaged in school by their SR and social and relational risk status. Notes. All prevalence rates are weighted to represent the US child population ages 3 to 17 years. aORs are adjusted for age, sex, race/ethnicity, income and insurance coverage type. [a]aORs are statistically significant after adjusting for age, sex, race/ethnicity, income and insurance coverage type. See Technical Appendix D1 for regression details associated with this figure.

in **Fig. 3**, across all SHR/RHR subgroups, the aORs that a child would more consistently demonstrate good SR skills were 3.44 to 10.04 times greater for children with stronger PCC compared to those with poorer PCC. In turn, better SR is associated with improved school-related outcomes as noted earlier.

Notably, the prevalence of children with MEB whose families consistently practiced resilience skills was generally lower than for those without MEB (29.4% vs 38.7%, $P<.001$), but was not high for either group (see **Table 1**). Variation in this prevalence across the 4 SHR/RHR subgroups of children with MEB ranged from 22.7% to 35.9% ($P<.001$). The prevalence of children with MEB who experienced stronger PCC showed wider variation across SHR/RHR subgroups (40.6%–60.0%, $P<.001$). The aORs that a child experienced stronger PCC were 18% lower for children with SHR only, 48% lower for those with RHR only, and 55% lower for those with both SHR and RHR compared to children experiencing neither type of risk. See Appendix E1 for further details.

LIMITATIONS

This study has several limitations. First, analyses used cross-sectional data, preventing confirmation of causal relationships between US children's social and relational risks, protective family factors, and study outcomes. Yet, the NSCH provides

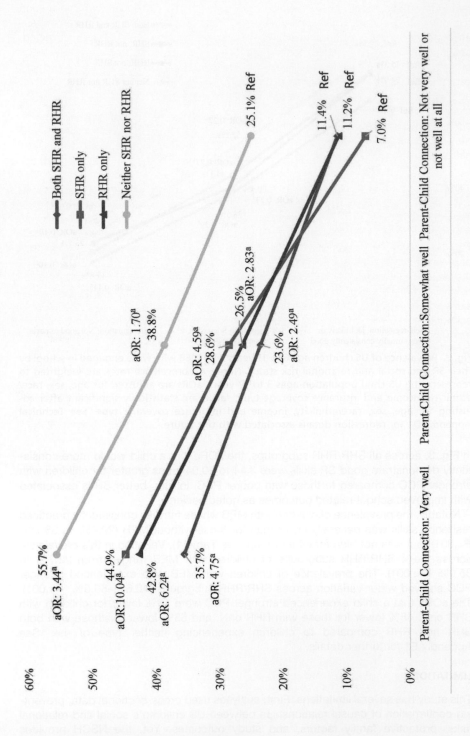

important population-based information and measurement generalizability that generate epidemiologic insights which are not feasible to do longitudinally on such a large scale. Second, findings may underestimate the prevalence of children experiencing social and/or RHR because: (1) measures represented higher levels of risk (eg, children with 2+ ACEs); and (2) positive caregiver reporting bias may lower prevalence of risks.[54,57] Third, measures of SR and PCC each rely on a single item. Findings might vary if additional measures of these constructs were included. We hypothesize that adding additional indicators would strengthen associations found in this study, especially for the "missed school" and "bullying victimization and/or perpetration" outcomes where associations with SR by SHR and RHR were weaker, suggesting it may be important to examine other aspects of SR related to internalizing versus externalizing reactions to social and relational stress for children.

DISCUSSION

This study documents a 21.8% prevalence of MEB among US children that varies 4-fold, from 15.1% to 60.4%, based on the SHR and/or RHR children experience (see **Fig. 1**). Over two-thirds (67.6%) of US children with MEB experienced one or more of the evidence-based social and/or RHR evaluated. This prevalence is notable given that study SHR and RHR indices identified children with serious, rather than minimal, risks. Children with MEB and any SHR and/or RHR were less likely to demonstrate SR skills and engage in school and were more likely to both miss more than 2 weeks of school in a year and have been a victim and/or perpetrator of bullying at school. Offering hope, children with MEB were more likely to demonstrate good SR skills if their family reported consistently practicing resilience skills and had a stronger PCC. These protective factors are malleable and can be promoted using evidence-based strategies.[14,66–68] As we show here, doing so is expected to also increase school engagement and reduce missed school days and bullying victimization and perpetration among children with MEB.

Understanding the full population prevalence of the SHR and RHR associated with MEB is important for determining whether to advance high-risk versus population-wide efforts to assess and reduce these risks among US children, ideally before they manifest as symptoms that may lead to an MEB diagnosis. In this study, we found that nearly half of US children without MEB also experienced SHR and/or RHR (49.3%) and that RHR were the most common type of risk for children whether they had MEB or not. Similarly, associations found between improved SR and improved school engagement for children with MEB across all SHR or RHR subgroups were also found for children without MEB (see Appendix C1). These results suggest that population-wide efforts are needed to both assess and reduce RHR, along with SHR, and to promote SR and positive mental health among all US children and their families.

Although evaluated at a national level here, findings can be generated for all US states with the combined years NSCH data used in this study. State-level findings

◄───

Fig. 3. Prevalence of US children ages 6 to 17 years who demonstrate SR ("definitely true" or "always/usually"), by their parent-child connection status (how well share/what really matters) and their social and RHR status. Data: 2016 to 2019 National Survey of Children's Health. Notes. All prevalence rates are weighted to represent the US child population ages 6 to 17 years. aORs are adjusted for age, sex, race/ethnicity, income and insurance coverage type. [a]aORs are statistically significant after adjusting for age, sex, race/ethnicity, income and insurance coverage type. See **Table 4** for confidence intervals for aORs.

can inform efforts like the current Integrated Care for Kids (InCK) state demonstrations[69] on the use of approaches to pay for health services for children taking into account SDOH.[70] Our findings support these and related efforts to promote a whole-child, whole-family assessment of both SHR and RHR, as well as strengths (SR, family resilience, PCC) experienced by children and families. Doing so can better inform the specification of prevention, diagnostic and treatment strategies to ensure that these efforts address the root causes of child mental health problems, like the toxic stress and trauma that can arise with the RHR and SHR evaluated here.[6] InCK and other related government and private sector children's health care (including mental health) payment innovations increasingly focus on implementing "value-based care."[71,72] This study suggests that these types of payment reforms must reflect the fact that most children and youth with MEB also experience SHR and RHR and may require different and more complex, cross-agency and integrated community-based approaches to promote positive outcomes.[73,74]

Findings also urge the continued scaling of family-centered, primary care medical homes that integrate mental health promotion and treatment capacities[6,75] and embrace the profound importance of children's social and relational environments, including child's/family's relationship with their health care teams.[6,26,76] Child health professionals are essential to help families learn and practice resilience skills and establish and maintain safe and strong nurturing connections with their children. This study demonstrates that doing so will improve SR and school and social outcomes even among children with MEB with higher levels of SHR and RHR. Promoting family, parenting, and child strengths even amid adversity requires multigenerational approaches that gain the trust and engagement of families as well as skills to build healing partnerships that nurture family protective factors.[6,75–79] This may result in a greater sense of positive impact among child health professionals and, in turn, lead to much needed improvements in their joy and satisfaction in their work.[78]

Investments are required to build the knowledge, skills, and capacity of child mental health and primary care professionals as well as school and other community-based professionals who must work together to promote positive mental health for children.[5,6,74] It is especially important to disseminate information across all child-serving professionals and agencies about approaches to (1) increase PCC and family resilience; (2) recognize and improve children's SR and other resiliency skills; and (3) implement evidence-based clinical and public health approaches to prevent, mitigate impacts of and heal developmental trauma. Doing so will require shifting focus away from diagnosis of discrete child mental health symptoms to a primary focus on promoting positive relational health within the lives of children and development of their social and emotional skills.[6,26] Science is strong that when relational health is compromised or undeveloped, children can experience a myriad of symptoms associated with common mental health diagnoses. For instance, the symptom of dissociation is a symptom associated with many children mental health problems, like depression, anxiety, and ADHD. Recognition that this symptom can be an adaptive coping response to relational poverty and/or abuse in the home will shift the focus to assessing and promoting relational health in the family and helping children heal and restore connection to their sensations and emotions and develop social and emotional skills needed to restore their functioning. Similarly, many children exposed to toxic stress and trauma related to the SHR and RHR they experience may adapt and cope by presenting as "normal" and even highly resilient, when in fact they have physiologic and more nuanced mental health symptoms indicative of toxic stress. These children also require support to promote their relational health in the family and to reduce sources of social stress that can also contribute to these RHR, like food insecurity and unsafe neighborhoods.[80]

Empowering communities to identify the risks, needs, priorities and strengths of their children, families, and young people is critical to ensure that both clinical and public health strategies are culturally appropriate and aligned with community values and priorities. Communities that Care (CTC) and Promoting School-University Partnerships to Enhance Resilience (PROSPER) are examples of community-engaged strategies in which researchers provide guidance to community coalitions in conducting assessments, identifying key risk and protective factors for youth in the community, and implementing evidence-based prevention programs at the school, family, and community levels to address youth issues prioritized by the community. CTC and PROSPER have each produced positive and sustained effects on youth health and well-being.[81–86] Few US communities, however, are currently engaged in these types of prevention initiatives. Widespread engagement of community stakeholders, including youth themselves, to identify locally relevant SHR and RHR and protective factors and implement evidence-informed interventions has potential to shift youth outcomes at a population level.

This study adds to the growing empirical evidence demonstrating that social and relational contexts are critical drivers of child mental health and functioning. We cannot hope to heal the large numbers of mental health challenges our children are experiencing and promote positive mental health with only a disease-oriented focus on treatment and addressing individual-level etiologic factors. Rather, a public health lens and social-ecological frame are needed to guide broad-based promotion, prevention, and treatment strategies that proactively support positive child and family mental health for all children and address root causes of child mental health problems when they occur. Such a preventative, healing-centered, and trauma-informed approach holds great promise to improve the health of children in the United States and the adults they will become.[6,14,26,87]

FUNDING SOURCE

Robert Wood Johnson Foundation, grant #75448 to Johns Hopkins Bloomberg School of Public Health (PI: Bethell).

DISCLOSURE

The authors have nothing to disclose.

REFERENCES

1. Leeb RT, Bitsko RH, Radhakrishnan L, et al. Mental health–related emergency department visits among children aged< 18 years during the COVID-19 pandemic—United States, January 1–October 17, 2020. Morb Mortal Weekly Rep 2020;69(45):1675.

2. Raviv T, Warren CM, Washburn JJ, et al. Caregiver perceptions of children's psychological well-being during the COVID-19 pandemic. JAMA Netw Open 2021; 4(4):e2111103.

3. Yard E, Radhakrishnan L, Ballesteros MF, et al. Emergency department visits for suspected suicide attempts among persons aged 12–25 years before and during the COVID-19 pandemic — United States, January 2019–May 2021. MMWR Morb Mortal Wkly Rep 2021;70(24):888–94.

4. Brown J. Children's Hospital Colorado declares mental health state of emergency as suicide attempts rise Suicide attempts are rising and emergency room visits for mental health crises were up 90% last month. Mental health experts are asking for help 2021. Available at: https://coloradosun.com/2021/05/25/mental-health-emergency-children-teen-colorado/. Accessed November 6, 2021.

5. Boat TF, Kelleher KJ. Fostering healthy mental, emotional, and behavioral development in child health care. JAMA Pediatr 2020;174(8):745–6.

6. Garner AS, Yogman M, the American Academy of Pediatrics Committee on Psychosocial Aspects of Child and Family Health, the Section on Developmental and Behavioral Pediatrics, and the Council on Early Childhood. Preventing childhood toxic stress: partnering with families and communities to promote relational health. Pediatrics 2021;148(2). e2021052582.

7. Black MM, Behrman JR, Daelmans B, et al. The principles of Nurturing Care promote human capital and mitigate adversities from preconception through adolescence. BMJ Glob Health 2021;6:e004436.

8. Gleason MM, Goldson E, Yogman M. The council on early childhood, the committee on psychosocial aspects of child and family health, and the section on developmental and behavioral pediatrics of the American Academy of pediatrics. Addressing early childhood emotional and behavioral problems. Pediatrics 2016;138(6):e20163025.

9. American Academy of Pediatrics Council on Community Pediatrics, Committee on Nutrition. Promoting food scurity for all children pediatrics. Pediatrics; 2015. p. 2015–3301.

10. Hatem C, Lee CY, Zhao X, et al. Food insecurity and housing instability during early childhood as predictors of adolescent mental health. J Fam Psychol 2020;34(6):721–30.

11. Fowler PJ, Farrell AF. Housing and child well being: implications for research, policy, and practice. Am J Community Psychol 2017;60(1–2):3–8.

12. James S, Donnelly L, Brooks-Gunn J, et al. Links between childhood exposure to violent contexts and Risky adolescent health behaviors. J Adolesc Health 2018; 63(1):94–101.

13. Trent M, Dooley DG, Dougé J. The impact of racism on child and adolescent health. Pediatrics 2019;144(2):e20191765.

14. Center on the Developing Child at Harvard University. Three principles to improve outcomes for children and families, 2021 update 2021. Available at: http://www.developingchild.harvard.edu. Accessed April 25, 2021 at 3Principles_Update2021v2.pdf.

15. Baldari C, Mathur R. Study shows Americans agree: poor child well-being is a top issue. First Focus. 2017. Available at: https://firstfocus.org/blog/most-americans-see-child-poverty-as-top-concern-study-finds. Accessed April 25, 2021.

16. Perrin JM, Duncan G, Diaz A, et al. Principles and policies to strengthen child and adolescent health and well-being: study describes national academies of sciences, engineering, and medicine reports on poverty, mental, emotional, and behavioral health, adolescence, and young family health and education. Health Aff 2020;39(10):1677–83.

17. McCabe MA, Leslie L, Counts N, et al. Pediatric integrated primary care as the foundation for healthy development across the lifespan. Clin Pract Pediatr Psychol 2020;8(3):278–87.

18. Seifert R, Deignan J. Transforming pediatrics to support population health. Farmington, CT: Child Health Development Institute; 2019.

19. Pascoe JM, Wood DL, Duffee JH, et al. Mediators and adverse effects of child poverty in the United States. Pediatrics 2016;137(4):e20160340.
20. Oh DL, Jerman P, Silvério Marques S, et al. Systematic review of pediatric health outcomes associated with childhood adversity. BMC Pediatr 2018;18(1):83.
21. Bethell CD, Newacheck P, Hawes E, et al. Adverse childhood experiences: assessing the impact on health and school engagement and the mitigating role of resilience. Health Aff (Millwood) 2014;33(12):2106–15.
22. Neece CL, Green SA, Baker BL. Parenting stress and child behavior problems: a transactional relationship across time. Am J Intellect Dev Disabil 2012;117(1): 48–66.
23. Schieve L, Boulet S, Kogan M, et al. Parenting aggravation and autism spectrum disorders: 2007 National Survey of Children's Health. Disabil Health J 2011;4: 143–52.
24. Mestre JM, Núñez-Lozano JM, Gómez-Molinero R, et al. Emotion regulation ability and resilience in a sample of adolescents from a suburban area. Front Psychol 2017;8:1980.
25. Lawson GM, McKenzie ME, Becker KD, et al. The core components of evidence-based social emotional learning programs. Prev Sci 2019;20:457–67.
26. Heller L, LaPierre A. Healing developmental trauma: how early trauma affects self-regulation, self-image, and the capacity for relationship. Berkeley, CA: North Atlantic Books; 2012.
27. Khanlou N, Wray R. A whole community approach toward child and youth resilience promotion: a review of resilience literature. Int J Ment Health Addict 2014;12(1):64–79.
28. Halpern J, Jutte D, Colby J, et al. Social dominance, school bullying, and child health: what are our ethical obligations to the very young? Pediatrics 2015; 135(Suppl 2):S24–30.
29. García-Carrión R, Villarejo-Carballido B, Villardón-Gallego L. Children and adolescents mental health: a systematic review of interaction-based interventions in schools and communities. Front Psychol 2019;10:918.
30. Housman DK. The importance of emotional competence and self-regulation from birth: a case for the evidence-based emotional cognitive social early learning approach. Int J Child Care Educ Policy 2017;11:13.
31. Pandey A, Hale D, Das S, et al. Effectiveness of Universal self-regulation-based interventions in children and adolescents: a systematic review and meta-analysis. JAMA Pediatr 2018;172(6):566–75.
32. Bronson MB. Recognizing and supporting the development of self-regulation in young children. Young Child 2000;32–7.
33. Yule K, Houston J, Grych J. Resilience in children exposed to violence: a meta-analysis of protective factors across ecological contexts. Clin Child Fam Psychol Rev 2019;22(3):406–31.
34. Fritz J, de Graaff AM, Caisley H, et al. A systematic review of amenable resilience factors that moderate and/or mediate the relationship between childhood adversity and mental health in young people. Front Psychiatry 2018;9:230.
35. Foster CE, Horwitz A, Thomas A, et al. Connectedness to family, school, peers, and community in socially vulnerable adolescents. Child Youth Serv Rev 2017; 81:321–31.
36. Bariola E, Gullone E, Hughes EK. Child and adolescent emotion regulation: the role of parental emotion regulation and expression. Clin Child Fam Psychol Rev 2011;14(2):198–212.

37. Allison MA, Attisha E, Council on School Health. The link between school attendance and good health. Pediatrics 2019;143(2):e20183648.

38. Arseneault L, Bowes L, Shakoor S. Bullying victimization in youths and mental health problems: 'much ado about nothing'? Psychol Med 2010;40(5):717–29.

39. Bethell CD, Jones J, Gombojav N, et al. Positive childhood experiences and adult mental and relational health in a statewide sample: associations across adverse childhood experiences levels. JAMA Pediatr 2019;173(11):e193007.

40. Bethell CD, Gombojav N, Whitaker R. Family resilience and connection promote flourishing among US children, even amid adversity. Health Aff 2019;38(5): 729–37.

41. Chen Y, Kubzansky L, VanderWeele T. Parental warmth and flourishing in mid-life. Soc Sci Med 2019;220:65–72.

42. O'Farrelly C, Watt H, Babalis D, et al. A brief home-based parenting intervention to reduce behavior problems in young children: a pragmatic randomized clinical trial. JAMA Pediatr 2021;175(6):567–76.

43. Kuhn ES, Laird RD. Family support programs and adolescent mental health: review of evidence. Adolesc Health Med Ther 2014;5:127–42.

44. Flouri E, Midouhas E, Joshi H, et al. Emotional and behavioural resilience to multiple risk exposure in early life: the role of parenting. Eur child Adolesc Psychiatry 2015;24(7):745–55.

45. Cates CB, Weisleder A, Berkule Johnson S, et al. Enhancing parent talk, Reading, and play in primary care: sustained impacts of the video interaction project. J Pediatr 2018;199:49–56 e41.

46. Suh B, Luthar SS. Parental aggravation may tell more about a child's mental/behavioral health than Adverse Childhood Experiences: using the 2016 National Survey of Children's Health. Child Abuse Negl 2020;101:104330.

47. Uddin J, Alharbi N, Uddin H, et al. Parenting stress and family resilience affect the association of adverse childhood experiences with children's mental health and attention-deficit/hyperactivity disorder. J Affect Disord 2020;272:104–9.

48. Ghandour RM, Jones JR, Lebrun-Harris LA, et al. The design and implementation of the 2016 national survey of children's health. Matern Child Health J 2017.

49. Child and Adolescent Health Measurement Initiative (CAHMI). 2016-2017 and 2018-2019 national survey of children's health SPSS codebooks, version 1.0. 2018 and 2021. Child and Adolescent Health Measurement Initiative.

50. Dong Y, Peng C-YJ. Principled missing data methods for researchers. SpringerPlus 2013;2:222.

51. Bethell, CD, Garner, AS, Blackwell, CK, et al. Technical Appendix: Social and Relational Health Risks and Common Mental Health Problems US Children. Available at: https://nam11.safelinks.protection.outlook.com/?url=https%3A%2F%2Fwww.cahmi.org%2Fdocs%2Fdefault-source%2Fdefault-document-library%2Fchild-adol-psych-paper-technical-appendices_june-2021.pdf%3Fsfvrsn%3D92d32364_0&data=04%7C01%7Cj.surendrakumar%40elsevier.com%7C84e84a99c5de4f4ece6c08d987349bf5%7C9274ee3f94254109a27f9fb15c10675d%7C0%7C0%7C637689482482822864%7CUnknown%7CTWFpbGZsb3d8eyJWIjoiMC4wLjAwMDAiLCJQIjoiV2luMzIiLCJBTiI6Ik1haWwiLCJXVCI6Mn0%3D%7C3000&sdata=xNHRsou36zNvGIlZYS8VNaVvuU1lAHyPjTA9bgF%2FbdU%3D&reserved=0.

52. Bethell CD, Blumberg SJ, Stein RE, et al. Taking stock of the CSHCN screener: a review of common questions and current reflections. Acad Pediatr 2015;15(2): 165–76.

53. Sameroff A, Seifer R, Barocas R, et al. Intelligence quotient scores of 4-year-old children: social-environmental risk factors. Pediatrics 1987;79(3):343–50.
54. Sameroff AJ, Seifer R, McDonough SC. Contextual contributors to the assessment of infant mental health. In: DelCarmen-Wiggins R, Carter A, editors. Handbook of infant, toddler, and preschool mental health assessment. New York, NY: Oxford University Press; 2004. p. 61–76.
55. Billioux A, Verlander K, Anthony S, et al. Standardized screening for health-related social needs in clinical settings: the accountable health communities screening tool. NAM Perspect 2017.
56. Dubowitz H. The safe environment for every kid model: promotion of children's health, development, and safety, and prevention of child neglect. Ped Ann 2014;43(11):e271–7.
57. MacCallum RC, Zhang S, Preacher KJ, et al. On the practice of dichotomization of quantitative variables. Psychol Methods 2002;7:19–40.
58. McDowell I. Measuring health: a guide to rating scales and Questionnaires. 3rd edition. New York: Oxford University Press; 2006.
59. Levinson D, Kaplan G. What does self rated mental health represent. J Public Health Res 2014;3(3):287.
60. Cohen J. Statistical power analysis for the behavioral sciences. 2nd edition. Hillsdale, NJ: Erlbaum; 1988.
61. Bethell CD, Carle A, Hudziak J, et al. Methods to assess adverse childhood experiences of children and families: toward approaches to promote child well-being in policy and practice. Acad Pediatr 2017;17(7):S51–69.
62. Phua DY, Kee MZL, Meaney MJ. Positive maternal mental health, parenting, and child development. Biol Psychiatry 2020;87(4):328–37.
63. Leis JA, Heron J, Stuart EA, et al. Associations between maternal mental health and child emotional and behavioral problems: does prenatal mental health matter? J Abnorm Child Psychol 2014;42(1):161–71.
64. Zhang S, Dang R, Yang N, et al. Effect of caregiver's mental health on early childhood development across different Rural communities in China. Int J Environ Res Public Health 2018;15(11):2341.
65. Moore KA, Bethell CD, Murphy D, et al. Flourishing from the start: what it is and how it can be measures. Child Trends 2017. Available at: https://www.childtrends.org/publications/flourishing-start-can-measured. Accessed November 5, 2020.
66. Hagan J, Shaw J, Duncan P. Bright futures: guidelines for health supervision of infants, children, and adolescents. 4th edition. Elk Grove Village: American Academy of Pediatrics; 2017.
67. Leslie LK, Mehus CJ, Hawkins JD, et al. Primary health care: potential home for family-focused preventive interventions. Am J Prev Med 2016;51(4 Suppl 2):S106.
68. Traub F, Boynton-Jarrett R. Modifiable resilience factors to childhood adversity for clinical pediatric practice. Pediatrics 2017;139(5):e20162569.
69. Alley DE, Ashford NC, Gavin AM. Payment innovations to drive improvements in pediatric care—the integrated care for Kids model. JAMA Pediatr 2019;173(8):717–8.
70. Newman N, Ferguson M, Dutton MJ, et al. In Pursuit of Whole Person Health: a review of social determinants of health (SDOH) initiatives in Medicaid managed care contracts and 1115 waivers. New York, NY: Manatt, Phelps, & Phillips, LLP; 2020.
71. Counts NZ, Roiland RA, Halfon N. Proposing the ideal alternative payment model for children. JAMA Pediatr 2021.

72. Mann C, Eder J. Don't Forget the Kids: care transformations that meet the needs of children. Acad Pediatr 2019;19(8):865–7.
73. Mann C, Ferguson M. Caring for the whole child: a new way to finance initiatives to improve children's health and well-being. Issue brief. New York, NY: Manatt, Phelps & Phillips, LLP; 2020.
74. Bethell CD, Kennedy S, Martinez-Vidal E, et al. Payment for progress: investing to catalyze child and family well-being using personalized and integrated strategies to address social and emotional determinants of health. CHA; 2018. Available at: https://academyhealth.org/sites/default/files/payment_for_progress_fullreport_nov2018.pdf. Accessed August 12, 2020.
75. Burkhart K, Asogwa K, Muzaffar N, et al. Pediatric integrated care models: a systematic review. Clin Pediatr (Phila) 2020;59(2):148–53.
76. Haine-Schlagel R, Walsh NE. A review of parent participation engagement in child and family mental health treatment. Clin Child Fam Psychol Rev 2015; 18(2):133–50.
77. Marsac ML, Kassam-Adams N, Hildenbrand AK, et al. Implementing a trauma-informed approach in pediatric health care networks. JAMA Pediatr 2016; 170(1):70–7.
78. Foy JM, Green CM, Earls MF, Committee on psychosocial aspects of child and family health, mental health leadership work group. Mental health competencies for pediatric practice. Pediatrics 2019;144(5):e20192757.
79. Gosar D, Košmrlj L, Musek PL, et al. Adaptive skills and mental health in children and adolescents with neuromuscular diseases. Eur J Paediatr Neurol 2021;30: 134–43.
80. McCrory EJ, Gerin MI, Viding E. Annual research review: childhood maltreatment, latent vulnerability and the shift to preventative psychiatry - the contribution of functional brain imaging. J Child Psychol Psychiatry 2017;58(4):338–57.
81. Brody GH, Yu T, Beach SR. Resilience to adversity and the early origins of disease. Dev Psychopathol 2016;28(4pt2):1347–65.
82. Oesterle S, Hawkins JD, Kuklinksi MR, et al. Effects of communities that care on males' and females' drug use and delinquency 9 years after baseline in a community-randomized trial. Am J Community Psychol 2015;56(3–4):217–28.
83. Oesterle S, Kuklinski MR, Hawkins JD, et al. Long-term effects of the communities that care trial on substance use, antisocial behavior, and violence through age 21 years. Am J Public Health 2018;108(5):659–65.
84. Spoth RL, Redmond C, Shin C, et al. PROSPER community-university partnership delivery system effects on substance misuse through 6 1/2 years past baseline from a cluster randomized controlled intervention trial [published erratum appears in Prev Med. 2014;69:36]. Prev Med 2013;56(3–4):190–6.
85. Rhew IC, Hawkins JD, Murray DM, et al. Evaluation of community-level effects of communities that cARE on adolescent drug use and delinquency using a repeated cross-sectional design. Prev Sci 2016;17(2):177–87.
86. Hawkins JD, Oesterle S, Brown EC, et al. Youth problem behaviors 8 years after implementing the communities that care prevention system: a community randomized trial. JAMA Pediatr 2014;168(2):122–9.
87. Kim BK, Gloppen KM, Rhew IC, et al. Effects of communities that care prevention system on youth reports of protective factors. Prev Sci 2015;16(5):652–62.

#KidsAnxiety and the Digital World

Jenna Glover, PhD[a,b], Merlin Ariefdjohan, PhD, MPH[b], Sandra L. Fritsch, MD, MSEd[a,b],*

KEYWORDS

- Child anxiety • Adolescent anxiety • Social media • Internet • Online gaming
- Digital technology

KEY POINTS

- Currently, there is limited research guiding clinicians' understanding of child or adolescent anxiety and the negative and positive impact social media may have on youth with anxiety.
- Problematic internet use in children and adolescents adversely affects sleep and healthy living habits (eg, diet, physical activity, sun exposure) that may exacerbate anxiety and depression.
- Limitations in research include potential biases toward negative consequences of digital technology and youth.
- There are emerging prevention and treatment tools through eHealth and mHealth technologies for addressing childhood anxiety.
- Recent COVID-19 restrictions and increased virtual platforms for education, meeting basic needs, and socialization are leading to "new norms" with respect to youth and screen time.

INTRODUCTION

Anxiety is the most common mental health condition in childhood, with prevalence rates ranging from 5% to 10% in children and up to 25% in teens.[1,2] When "screens" were first introduced through network television in the 1950s, children and teens may have seen 30 minutes of informational content on the national nightly news. Now anyone connected to the internet has access to constant streaming of news for 24 hours a day. Pandemic-related lockdowns, changing to virtual platforms for education, and an abrupt change of the social fabric for children and youth of all ages have led to an increase in prevalence of anxiety since March 2020.[3–5] Untreated anxiety in

[a] Pediatric Mental Health Institute, Children's Hospital Colorado, 13123 East 16th Avenue, B130, Aurora, CO 80045, USA; [b] Department of Psychiatry, University of Colorado Anschutz Medical Campus, 13001 East 17th Place, F546, Aurora, CO 80045, USA
* Corresponding author. Pediatric Mental Health Institute, Children's Hospital Colorado, 13123 East 16th Avenue, B130, Aurora, CO 80045.
E-mail address: Sandra.Fritsch@childrenscolorado.org

Child Adolesc Psychiatric Clin N Am 31 (2022) 71–90
https://doi.org/10.1016/j.chc.2021.06.004
1056-4993/22/© 2021 Elsevier Inc. All rights reserved.

childpsych.theclinics.com

youth can lead to other mental health conditions, including depression and substance use disorders. Common presentations of anxiety in younger children include fear of separation from a caregiver, social worries, specific phobias, and anxiety with novel situations. Typically, a child's world is filled with developmental social tasks that are potentially anxiety provoking (eg, separating from parents to attend school, making friendships and managing peer relationships, learning, active class participation, and pursuing interests or socializing beyond the school setting). In adolescence, developing complex peer relationships, including romantic relationships, as well as planning for adulthood can cause or exacerbate anxiety. Over the past 10 years, social media and digital technology have become prominent components of our youth's lives, with usage peaking among 16- to 24-year-olds.[6] Younger children are also increasingly exposed to the digital world and social media.

This article reviews current understanding of how childhood anxiety disorders interplay with electronic media, including risks and protective factors, challenges faced by caretakers navigating the digital world of youth, and current and potential future digital apps ("apps") to treat anxiety in children and adolescents. This article includes the impact of the coronavirus disease 2019 (COVID-19) pandemic on child mental health, screen time, and preparing for a "new norm" for our youth and digital technology.

RISK FACTORS ASSOCIATED WITH COMPUTER HABITS

The ubiquitous nature of digital technology in the everyday life of modern youth makes it essential for clinicians to understand the potential risks these mediums pose. The currently limited research on the relationship between technology and anxiety in children and adolescents suggests there are associations between computer habits and symptoms of anxiety.[7–12] To best understand the implications of these relationships, the following are important:

1. Understand how the developmental tasks of youth are affected by technology habits.
2. Recognize how digital communication differs from face-to face interactions for anxious youth.
3. Identify individual factors associated with anxiety and problematic internet use (PIU) in youth.
4. Examine unique features of social media that may serve to worsen anxiety in young people.

Developmental Tasks

One of the major tasks of childhood and adolescence is the creation and maintenance of significant relationships. Friendship in childhood is followed by increasingly intimate relationships in adolescence. Modern life has changed the nature of play in the lives of youth. Most parents no longer consider wandering local neighborhoods to be safe for their children, thus virtual worlds provide an alternate setting for play.[13] The COVID-19 pandemic that led to lockdowns, social distancing, and virtual schooling throughout 2020 to 2021 has impacted developmental tasks of childhood and adolescence.[14] Conversely, the sense of safety provided by the digital world has enabled shy youth to explore friendships in games geared toward children as young as 5 years old. Games and websites, such as Fortnite, Roblox, Terraria, and Zuluworld, are developed for younger children and allow limited social networking.[15] Grom Social is a social networking site for children aged 10 years and older, which has been described as safe but turns out to be flawed because links sometimes lead to inappropriate sites.[15] YouTube Kids has been marketed for youth as young as 4 years of age, and Instagram is in the process of creating an Instagram platform for those younger than age thirteen.[16] Minecraft is a popular video game played by latency-aged children that can facilitate engagement with peers in person and virtually.[17] Despite the growing number of these platforms, there is little research evidence to date regarding the potential of social media to facilitate friendships in younger children. Inherent risks of heavy digital technology engagement for latency-age anxious children include sleep impairment, use of the virtual world to avoid normative exposures in the real world, inadequate exercise, and development of problematic overuse.[18-20]

Important milestones of adolescence include the development of identity and managing relationships with peers. Self-presentation is the process by which individuals selectively manage the image and identity shown to others. Self-disclosure involves sharing one's thoughts, feelings, and behaviors.[21] Both self-presentation and self-disclosure are critical in the exploration of identity and relationships with others. However, anxiety may interfere with an adolescent's self-presentation efficacy, leading to avoidance of social interactions with peers. Thus, computer-mediated communication (CMC) offers an alternative platform to engage with others that is typically perceived by socially anxious youth as safer than face-to-face contact.

Computer-Mediated Communication

Social anxiety involves the fear of negative evaluation by others. Consequently, socially anxious youth tend to avoid experiences they believe may result in unfavorable impressions.[22] As CMC allows for text-based conversations without resorting to traditional audio or visual cues, this provides a comforting alternative for youth fearing judgements about their appearance, speech, and manifestation of physiologic signs of anxiety (eg, blushing).[23] CMC also enables asynchronized communication that allows participants to take more time to construct and edit messages before sending them. Asynchronicity especially appeals to youth who are self-conscious, easily embarrassed, or likely to withdraw in face-to-face settings.[21]

Social anxiety is positively related to preference for the freedom from nonverbal cues provided by CMC, according to a meta-analytic review of 22 studies.[23] The review found that socially anxious individuals prefer online interaction to in-person interaction and are more likely than peers to consider it as an effective medium for developing relationships.[23] With the greater comfort and perceived increased in self-presentational efficacy provided by CMC, the socially anxious individual's preference for online social interactions may be a risk factor for the development of PIU.[24]

Problematic Internet Use

PIU can lead to the development of cognitive and behavioral symptoms that result in distress and impairment in functioning.[22] PIU involves difficulty controlling the amount of time an individual spends online and distress when internet access is unavailable or poor bandwidth provides suboptimal virtual experiences.[23] PIU was one of the first and most broadly used terms in the taxonomy of tech-related problems and disorders. It has also been used interchangeably with other terms such as video game addiction (IVGA) or internet gaming disorder, internet addiction, virtual addiction, and technology addiction.

With the continued increase in different types of technologies, platforms, and use among youth as well as expanded research in these areas, several new terms have emerged in the literature identifying specific subcategories under the umbrella of PIU:

- "Appearance-related social media consciousness" is the extent to which individuals' thoughts and behaviors reflect ongoing awareness of whether they might look attractive to a social media audience. Such self-objectification tendencies have been associated with higher likelihood of anxiety as well as depression and eating disorders.[25]
- "Nomophobia" (ie, "no mobile phone") is the experience of extreme discomfort, anxiety, nervousness, or anguish caused by being out of contact with a mobile phone. Sharma and colleagues (2019) noted that this is an emerging mental health condition and is significantly associated with anxiety, depression, and poor quality of life.[26]
- "Phubbing" is a social exclusion behavior related to excessive focus on mobile phone use whereby an individual is being snubbed in favor of the phone (ie, phone snubbing). This habit can undermine interpersonal connection and have adverse effects to relationships that may subsequently affect mental health.[27] Of note, parents may feel "phubbed" by their child.
- "Social media disorder" (SMD) is a behavioral addiction where individuals experience uncontrollable urges to be on social media and to maintain an active presence in the platform at all times, as well as being overly concerned about the happenings in the social media and their perceived persona. The constant stream of approval in the form of retweet, likes, and shares from social media platforms induce dopamine that triggers the brain's reward area similar to those caused by other addictive agents including gambling and using recreation drugs.[28]

As the nomenclature grows under PIU, it is necessary for us to understand emergent information regarding prevalence and risk factors associated with these problem areas and their impact on young people. Various studies worldwide have noted that PIU results in impaired human interaction, poorer sleep quality, and development of unhealthy lifestyle habits (eg, less exercise, higher consumption of fast foods and sugary beverages, among others).[18-20,29-31] Furthermore, a history of psychological illness is associated with PIU. Users experiencing psychological problems may use online activity to escape negative feelings and increase positive ones, potentially creating a pattern of compulsive use.[7] Research has found that socially anxious youth needing social assurance are more likely to develop addiction to social media than those with little need for such assurance.[32] Socially anxious youth seeking to manage anxiety through external validation also seem to be at greater risk for developing problematic use than those with less need for social approval. These results reflect the importance of understanding individual cognitions and attitudes about online engagement because individuals are affected differently by internet habits.[33-35]

The type of screen time activity being used (active vs passive) can also be a risk factor for developing PIU. Active screen time is defined as time when an individual is actively engaging with the virtual platform such as learning skills, doing something creative, reading, or video chatting with another person. In contrast, passive screen time occurs when an individual is mindlessly scrolling through social media or watching TV or a movie. Passive screen time and the use of portable devices have been associated with higher likelihood of anxiety disorders and sleep disturbances.[19,20,36] Engagement in pathologic video gaming has also been identified as a risk factor in the development of anxiety in youth. In a longitudinal study, pathologic gaming (ie, use that disrupts interpersonal, psychological, and/or academic functioning) was noted to be a predictor for depression, anxiety, and social phobia. Children and adolescents who were able to stop pathologic gaming showed a reduction in all 3 areas compared with peers who remained pathologic gamers.[37] These results are notable because this is the first research demonstrating that pathologic gaming is predictive of later-onset and maintenance of mental health disorders.

Social Media and Anxiety

Social media sites are designed to allow users to share content, interact with others, and disseminate information about themselves and their world.[38] Numerous social media platforms are used by both children and adolescents (eg, Spotlite, PopJam, Instagram, Snapchat, YouTube, TikTok). Social media sites play an important role in self-presentation.[39] Platforms such as Facebook and Instagram allow users to develop a digital identity that can be carefully constructed and digitally enhanced to the point of idealization, potentially creating a culture of unrealistic comparisons. Many youths feel the need to be constantly connected to social media platforms to maintain a presence in their peer group and may use social networking sites to alleviate the fear of missing out (FOMO).

FOMO is worry about missing connections that peers are enjoying without you, potentially risking loss of social status. Youth indicate that FOMO often results in anxiety and feelings of inadequacy.[6] Anxious youth, who also have heightened FOMO, are more likely to experience problems in functioning related to their use of social media. High levels of FOMO in youth mediated the relationship between anxiety symptoms and negative consequences (eg, impairment in academic and/or social functioning).[7] Unlimited access to many idealized representations of peers via social media can lead youth to believe that peers are leading better, happier, and more fulfilled lives. This engenders anxiety, self-consciousness, and perfectionism, which subsequently triggers compulsive use of social networking sites.[6,40]

Maintaining multiple social media accounts simultaneously is commonplace among youth and has been positively correlated with anxiety.[38] Youth who operate multiple social media sites may feel social pressure to sustain a carefully crafted online identity on multiple fronts, resulting in preservative thoughts and behaviors. Engagement with multiple social media platforms also increases demands for multitasking, which has been found to worsen mood and anxiety.[38] Adolescents who habitually plug in to social media late at night displace much-needed sleep. One in 5 youth report waking during the night to check messages on social media.[6] Having multiple social media accounts seems to increase cognitive demands, impair restorative sleep, increase tendencies for forming obsessive internet habits, and increase risk for anxiety.[6]

Some youth use social media to avoid unpleasant emotions and real-world stressors through distraction, excessive viewing of others' social media profiles (eg, passively viewing Instagram profiles, known as Instastalk), or posting complaints. Lonely teens may use social media, a more comfortable mechanism for expression, as an emotion-regulation strategy.[7] Ohannessian and colleagues (2021) pointed out that excessive social media use also increases the likelihood of corumination (ie, repeatedly discussing personal problems with peers), which subsequently lead to internalizing problems and anxiety symptoms.[35] These factors can lead to PIU impairing real-world relationships, especially in lonely individuals who prefer socializing online.[22] Young people often use social media to gain relief from distress (eg, loneliness, anxiety), but overuse increases the risk of a cyclic pattern of avoidant coping and social isolation, addictive use of social media, and ultimately exacerbated loneliness and social anxiety[41,42] (**Fig. 1**). Research has underscored this risk, identifying that youth experiencing SMD have higher rates of loneliness and sleep problems and are more likely to experience ostracism in daily living.[28]

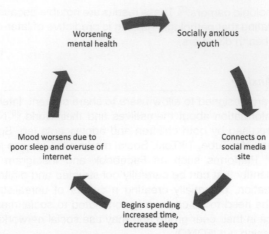

Fig. 1. Cycle of socially anxious youth and social media.

Limitations

Research in this area is continuing to develop but several limitations exist currently. First, most aforementioned studies are based on cross-sectional designs, of which causality is unclear.[38] For example, associations between anxiety and social media use may indicate that individuals with anxiety tend to use social media more, or that increased use of social media worsens anxiety, or both. Additional research using experimental design is needed to establish the direction of these relationships. Second, most studies have focused on older adolescents and young adults, so there is limited research on the relationship of social media use and anxiety among preadolescent children.[33] Third, most research is focused on community-based populations, and more work is needed studying these relationships in clinical populations.[38] Also of note, recent publications assessing/describing the impact of internet and social media use during the pandemic on pediatric mental health have been published at an exceptionally rapid pace in response to the pandemic. Many recent studies were limited to descriptive studies of a unique time and may not be generalizable to all post-pandemic settings.

BENEFITS AND PROTECTIVE FACTORS

There are several means by which online activities can benefit children and teens. The online world of youth is typically intertwined with their offline lives. Both can work in conjunction to support individual and interpersonal development.[39] Social media provides an opportunity for young people to share their own creations and demonstrate mastery: videos, pictures, blogs, and tweets. Status updates allow practice expressing self-disclosure skills, permitting communication that might otherwise be impossible. Social media is a platform for adolescent self-expression that can provide the framework for the development of identity while concurrently offers countless opportunities to connect with others of similar interests and enhance real-world social relationships.[6] Furthermore, preadolescents and adolescents interact online to remain connected to their real-world friends, which also confers important benefits for developing communication skills and maintaining interpersonal relationships.[33]

The internet also provides access to potential networks of support. Most teenagers surveyed endorsed having received support via social media during times of distress.[6] Online sources of support may be particularly helpful for youth whose anxiety interferes with their ability to seek support face-to-face. Specialized social media sites related to mental health (eg, Half of Us, Go Ask Alice!, To Write Love on Her Arms, Today is For Tomorrow, TeenMentalHealth.org) provide a platform for youth to access information and potential support from peers encountering similar problems, which may help alleviate stigma related to seeking help for mental health issues.[38] However, it is important for providers to understand how these sites operate and potential risks associated with the use of these sites.

Youth who are part of marginalized groups (eg, LGBTQIA youth) are at higher risk for developing mental health problems. They may find safety, support, and information through online interactions and social networking.[43] For example, nonheterosexual youth are able to connect, discuss aspects of identity, receive affirmation and support, and practice coming out.[21] Social media platforms also represent hubs of community for transgender adolescents. These communities provide emotional, appraisal, and informational support that transgender youth may not otherwise be able to access.[43] Research has found that adolescent mothers' use of social networking sites is related to reduced anxiety and improved confidence.[44] Given the potential of digital technology and platforms to support the most vulnerable youth, it is important that these youth are able to have access to these resources.[45] Without appropriate access to the internet, we are further exacerbating pre-existing disparities for our most vulnerable youth. An overview of risk and protective factors related to online engagement and anxiety is summarized in **Table 1**.

PARENTING AN ANXIOUS CHILD IN THE DIGITAL AGE

Children today are digital natives, whereas some parents are not. Parents may lack the technical abilities to keep pace with their childrens and may be unaware that passwords or filters are easily bypassed by savvy youth.[46] Parents and grandparents providing supervision are frequently naïve to the concept that children's offline lives intertwine with their online lives and that social media can also facilitate healthy socialization.[47] Managing the online behaviors of a socially anxious child is particularly challenging in balancing the need to limit the child's time spent online and protecting them from online risks with the potential benefits of increased socialization. Parents may also be prone to blame technology as the primary cause of mental health problems and be disconnected from younger generation's views of the vital role that technology and social media play in their lives.[45] Parents may struggle to reconcile this mixed picture, for example, when video games such as Minecraft are incorporated into school curricula, when providers recommend treatment applications ("apps") for anxiety, and when they may struggle with their own maladaptive internet habits.

Health care providers play a vital role in educating and guiding parents on the different ways that technology devices and platforms can impact child development in both positive and negative ways.[48] Providers need working knowledge and skills to support families as they navigate these complex issues. For example, youth may engage excessively with computers (eg, playing videogames) to avoid anxious thoughts, feelings, and physiologic symptoms that are triggered by real-world activities (eg, going to school, social activities with peers). When socially anxious youth refuse to go to in-person schooling (when available), caregivers should be advised to limit or restrict media and internet use until successful attendance occurs. Providers should advise caregivers to not allow youth with significant anxiety symptoms to

Table 1
Risk and benefits of online habits for youth with anxiety

Risks for Developing Problematic Internet Use/Consequences of PIU	Benefits of Online Engagement
History of premorbid mental health concerns	Identity exploration and expression
Loneliness	Practice with self-disclosure
Shyness	Increased creativity
Preference for online social interactions	Augmenting real-world social relationships
Great need for social assurance	Access to health-related information
High levels of Fear of Missing Out (FOMO)	Increased availability of mental health treatments
Use social media for more than 2 h daily	Destigmatizing mental health forums
Multiple social media accounts	Companionship for members of marginalized groups
Case Example 1: A 10-year-old with long history of anxiety; separation concerns, social phobia, generalized anxiety concerns has open access to constant news feed and recent mass shootings, COVID deaths, and natural disasters has led to further fears of leaving home and returning to school.	*Case Example 1:* A 13-year-old female adolescent always socially shy, able to connect with peers online to "practice" social conversations and engagement. Family monitors to ensure peers are "real peers", from school or extracurricular activities.
Case Example 2: A 14-year-old adolescent has been exploring sexuality and gender on the internet. Has been on Omegele and other sites for social connections. Felt "safe". Shared worries, concerns, and nude pictures online. Was "catfished" and then instructed to Venmo $2000 or nude photos would be posted on multiple social media platforms. Had panic attacks and became suicidal.	*Case Example 2:* An 8-year-old precocious boy teaching others on his YouTube channel about ways to overcome nervousness, speak up in class, make a new friend, strategies to "conquer worries".

participate in online schooling that provides no face-to-face peer interactions, when alternative in-person schooling options exist because this reinforces avoidant coping. For anxious youth, behavior plans that grant online entertainment as a positive reward for exposure to and engagement in real-world activities can promote the practice of active rather than avoidant coping. Finally, providers should consider the impact of caregiver mental health (and personal technology use) on children's use of technology because parents who experience long-standing distress may rely on the use of screens to help manage children resulting in less oversight of time on screens and the quality of content being viewed.[49]

PIU among mothers of young children has been associated with maternal social anxiety and a positive relationship between social media and social anxiety in offspring.[50] Maternal depression has also been associated with screen overuse among Korean children aged 2 to 5 years.[49]

Notably, there are several online resources that are available for managing children's and family's digital technology habits (**Table 2**).

Table 2 Resources for families		
Resource	Link to Resource	Potential Use
Facts for Families Guide by the American Academy of Child & Adolescent Psychiatry (AACAP)	https://www.aacap.org/aacap/families_and_youth/facts_for_families/fff-guide/FFF-Guide-Table-of-Contents.aspx	Downloadable materials to guide parents in matters related to social media and internet use, including documents titled "Internet Use in Children", "Listening to Music and Watching Music Videos", "Movies, Media, and Children", "News and Children", "Social Media and Teens", "TV Violence and Children", "Video Games and Children: Playing with Violence", and "Watching TV/Screen Time and Children"
Healthy Children.org website by the American Academy of Pediatrics (AAP)	https://www.healthychildren.org/English/family-life/Media/Pages/How-to-Make-a-Family-Media-Use-Plan.aspx	Practical guidelines and support for families around mindful media use from birth through adolescence
Age-Based Media Reviews for Families by Common Sense Media	https://www.commonsensemedia.org/	Guidelines for parents around media use, and independent ratings of appropriateness of social media apps and games for youth of various ages
The App Evaluation Model by the American Psychiatric Association (APA)	https://www.psychiatry.org/psychiatrists/practice/mental-health-apps/the-app-evaluation-model	Evaluation of mental health apps including ease of use, privacy and safety, clinical foundation, and therapeutic benefits.

SCREEN TIME AND ANXIETY

According to the American Academy of Child and Adolescent Psychiatry (AACAP), children aged 8 to 12 years are spending on average 4 to 6 hours per day online, and teens up to 9 hours per day; however, the World Health Organization recommends no screen time for less than 1 year of age, at most 1 hour for preschoolers, and no more than 2 hours per day for all other youth ("Screen Time and Children" in AACAP Facts for Families Guide; **Table 2**). A commentary was published describing concerns of increased screen exposure of 40% among toddlers younger than 2 years with a smart phone and the potential impact on attachment and the development self-soothing skills.[51] Most recently published stories about screen time use and mental health conditions in youth are reviews of previous studies and report a "weak effect" of higher screen time use (greater than 2 hours per day) and trend toward increased anxiety.[12,19,52] When teasing out differences between active and passive screen time, greater than 4 hours per day of passive screen time was associated with increased rates of generalized anxiety disorder and social phobia in Canadian youth aged 12 to 18 years.[36] Additionally, the 4th survey of the Childhood and Adolescence Surveillance and Prevention of Adult Non-Communicable Disease (CASPIAN-IV) study indicated that screen time greater than 2 hours per day was associated with less physical activity and an increase in anxiety among those aged 6 to 18 years.[18] In considering these findings, it is important to underscore that these studies are correlation studies that did not show causation. Furthermore, recent calls have been made to abandon the construct of screen time. Instead, perspectives should shift toward how youth are interacting with technology in their daily lives and the quality of these interactions rather than the quantity.[45]

TECHNOLOGY AND TREATMENT OF ANXIETY

Youth frequently use online searches and social networking to learn about health-related topics. Teens use online resources to gather health information, share their own related experiences, learn of others' experiences, and track data related to health goals.[53] Therapists have begun to use social networking, including the creation and posting of TikTok videos, to provide mental health literacy and help destigmatize mental illness and reach a broad audience of youth. Online platforms can also augment or replace conventional treatment. Mobile health (mHealth) interventions involve the use of text messaging and smart phone apps, whereas electronic health (eHealth) interventions include videogames and other computer-based interventions. Both mHealth and eHealth may augment conventional therapies or serve as stand-alone interventions for anxiety disorders and distress associated with medical procedures and conditions.[54]

There are numerous potential benefits offered by mHealth and eHealth interventions that can expand the scope of mental health services. Online treatments are often cost-effective and could increase accessibility for families with limited time, financial resources, transportation options, and who are in remote locations with few or no mental health care providers. They may also be preferable for anxious youth who desire greater autonomy and anonymity.[55] However, the efficacy of these novel treatments remains unproven, and when used in lieu of traditional care, they risk delaying access to more effective treatments.

Mobile Health Apps

Mental health care providers can partner with youth in using mHealth resources in a variety of ways.[56] Apps can be used to help youth better engage in treatment via reminders to take medication (eg, Round Health Medicine Reminder and Pill Tracker), track mood (eg, Moodtrack Diary), keep thought diaries (eg, Moodnotes Thought Journal), or engage in self-regulatory skills such as mindfulness (eg, Calm: Meditation to Relax, Focus & Sleep Better). A review report published in 2016 had cited 55 apps intended to help youth with anxiety available on Google Play and the Apple App store.[57]

Despite the availability of many mHealth interventions, there is limited research on the acceptability and usability of these apps and almost no research on the effectiveness of these apps. Bry and colleagues (2018) published an article reviewing 121 apps marketed to treat anxiety in youth.[58] The authors checked for the presence/absence of six evidence-based treatment (EBT) components: (1) psychoeducation, (2) self-monitoring, (3) cognitions and thought challenging, (4) problem-solving, (5) contingency management, (6) exposures. They also assessed for relaxation training. The content was at a 9th grade reading level. User safety was limited regarding confidentiality and risk statements leading to intervention. Only 23% of the apps reviewed contained at least two EBT components. The majority of the apps were distraction tools, games, coloring activities, and audio or visual distractions. About half provided relaxation strategies. The "Reach for Success" mental health application, which is a 6-session cognitive behavioral therapy (CBT)-based protocol designed for prevention of anxiety problems in children 8 to 12 years old, was one of the few that were examined for usability. Children and preadolescents rated the app as having high usability, but future research is needed determine its effectiveness.[59] Grist and colleagues (2017) reviewed 24 articles that reported on 15 mental health apps for adolescents.[60] Among those reviewed, only two apps included randomized control trials, and there was no evidence found supporting the effectiveness of apps designed for children or teens with mental health concerns.

Clinicians should be aware of the variety of risks related to the use of these apps and educate patients and families regarding their potential dangers. Reviews of apps currently marketed for youth experiencing anxiety and depression demonstrated problems including lack of validated screening tools, lack of information regarding screening results, and insufficient professional support for apps that track negative mood and thinking patterns.[61] There is also an increased risk of harm through viewing strong and triggering negative contents posted in apps with sharing features. Notably, most apps do not have safeguards to warn users about negative contents or other systems that flag users who post suicidal comments. A recent review of apps for depression observed that less than a quarter of apps provided access to immediate suicide prevention or online therapeutic helplines.[61] Other risks inherent in using these apps are related to confidentiality and privacy.[58] Most apps currently available do not address confidentiality and use inadequate password protection, which could lead to data breaches. They also tend not to inform users about the types of data being collected and how these are used by the developers, nor provide options for users to control their privacy setting.[58] These concerns highlight the importance of increasing regulations of mental health apps to improve their quality, as well as to further promote the safety of individuals that use these platforms particularly youth.[60]

Finally, there is significant gap between apps available on the marketplace for download and apps that have been developed and are being researched in academic settings.[60] Despite the potential benefits of apps in addressing anxiety (eg, delivering of empirically based treatments, tracking of symptoms using self-report and/or bio-data), it is important to recognize there is a gap in research to marketplace that needs to be addressed to effectively understand how mHealth interventions can and should be implemented among youth.[58] Considering that such minimal research validates the effectiveness of mental health apps for anxiety, providers should evaluate the content of individual apps before recommending use with patients. This kind of review is important given increasing numbers of youth are using apps and social networking sites to learn more about and gain support for their mental health.[62] To help assist with this process, the American Psychiatric Association has developed "The App Evaluation Model" which provides a hierarchical rating system to guide providers, parents, and patients in evaluating an app and how it may differ from traditional treatment modalities. The model includes a brief eight-question screener or the option for more comprehensive evaluation across five domains which include access and background, privacy and safety, clinical foundation, usability, and therapeutic goal.[63]

Electronic Health Prevention and Interventions

Other programs have also been developed for prevention and treatment of anxiety disorders in children and adolescents. Prevention programs have the potential to significantly reduce the burden of mental health problems for youth. One online prevention program was adapted from a manualized face-to-face version, targeting younger children at risk for developing anxiety disorders. Researchers conducted a randomized controlled trial comparing parents of inhibited preschoolers participating in an 8-module online prevention program providing psychoeducation and skills for anxiety reduction (The Cool Little Kids) to controls. Participants reported high rates of satisfaction, and the children in the intervention group showed significantly improved anxiety compared with controls.[55]

A growing number of online programs show promise in the treatment of anxiety disorders. Some are intended to augment face-to-face psychotherapy, and others are intended as stand-alone therapy. Examples include Fearfighter, Beating the Blues, and The Brave Program. Most use empirically supported CBT practices.[64] A review of randomized controlled trials for such programs found that internet-delivered CBT self-help programs were highly effective in treating children and adolescents with anxiety, yielding comparable adherence and outcomes as traditional psychotherapy.[64] Internet-based therapy research is continuing to grow and find promising results. A recent randomized clinical trial also found that internet-delivered CBT was efficacious for children and adolescents (aged 10–17 years) with social anxiety disorder.[65] Furthermore, a randomized clinical noninferiority trial comparison of internet-delivered CBT to in-person CBT for children and adolescents with obsessive compulsive disorder found that internet-delivered CBT (followed up by in-person CBT if necessary) resulted in noninferior difference in symptoms at the 6-month follow-up.[66] These encouraging results suggest that online CBT-based treatment programs may be a viable, affordable, and accessible option to treat youth with anxiety disorders.

Electronic Health and Anxiety Related to Other Health Conditions

There are several eHealth interventions to help with prevention and intervention of anxiety related to acute and chronic health conditions. Online programs and games have demonstrated effectiveness as tools for children with preoperative anxiety, anticipatory dental anxiety, and anxiety comorbid with chronic physical conditions.[67–70] Preoperative anxiety in children has been correlated with distress immediately after operation, after which maladaptive anxiety and poor functioning may persist for up to 2 weeks. Researchers have found that video game play significantly decreases perioperative anxiety, delirium, and time to discharge when compared with treatment as usual.[67,68]

Other eHealth interventions for youth with long-term physical conditions address anxiety related to illness or treatment. A qualitative study of eHealth for youth with chronic physical illnesses revealed "(1) chronic illness as an anxiety-provoking journey; (2) limited access to information and eHealth interventions to support the journey; and (3) desires (among patients and their families) for interventions that assist with better understanding of the illness, personal support, and peer connection (especially for illnesses that restrict contact such as cystic fibrosis)." Therefore, eHealth interventions such as Quest for the Code, Re-Mission, and SPARX may be particularly valuable.[69]

Finally, a review of 22 eHealth prevention and intervention studies for supporting mental health related to treatment of physical health found that studies using CBT had the highest portion of achieving at least one intended outcome (80%) compared with problem solving (71%) and education alone (60%) with the authors suggesting that modality needs to be selected based on the medical situation (eg, education may be more useful in preoperative situations and less helpful for chronic illness).[71] This review also found that 4 out of 5 intervention studies targeting anxiety were successful in reducing symptoms.[71] In general, eHealth interventions have significant potential to help youth facing acute and chronic illness to gain mental wellness and valuable knowledge, increase social support with peers with similar health conditions, and reduce anxiety associated with treatment.

COVID-19 PANDEMIC

The COVID-19 pandemic has impacted the lives of youth across the globe, disrupting all aspects of normalcy in day-to-day life and interfering with developmental tasks including educational progression and interpersonal maturation through social connectedness. The consequences of the pandemic and subsequent quarantines will likely be widespread and longstanding. Research on the impact of past quarantines has identified that quarantined youth experience higher rates of posttraumatic stress disorder, depression, anger, and anxiety and that these symptoms can be longstanding and pervasive.[72] Quarantines may also have differential impact based on age, with younger children demonstrating regressive and clingy behaviors whereas older children are more likely to become anxious, restless, angry, and withdrawn.[73]

Initial research on the COVID-19 pandemic indicates that youth mental health is being significantly impacted. In a study of three European countries conducted during the early phase of COVID-19, researchers found that parents commonly reported children feeling bored, irritable, lonely, restless, and anxious.[72] Anxiety continued to be a commonly reported symptom for children and teens throughout the pandemic with rates of anxiety doubling in youth compared with prepandemic levels.[74] Additionally, adolescents who had psychiatric disorders before the pandemic were likely more vulnerable to worsening and new symptoms due to disruptions in therapeutic care exacerbated by difficulties coping with confinement.[75] Faced with these obstacles, youth engaged in higher levels of screen time to cope and adjust to the changing landscape of life in a pandemic.[76]

The demands of the COVID-19 pandemic have highlighted both the benefits and risk of using technology to cope during distressing and crisis situations. With the loss of face-to-face interactions in real-life setting, virtual platforms including digital technology, social media, and interactive gaming serve as a way for peers to maintain connection and reduce the negative impacts of social isolation.[75] Additionally, social media provides an outlet for youth to express and process feelings related to the pandemic and to engage in self-expression and distraction activities. Despite these benefits, the increased screen time and social media use on youth included taking time away from engagement in healthy routines and behaviors (eg, sleep, diet, outdoor time, physical activity). Additionally, there is an unending amount of information available on the internet, which may or may not be factual, and large consumption of this information can lead to increased anxiety, depression, and confusion. Researchers examining usage and attitudes of social media during the pandemic found that youth were more likely to report social media as being more valuable and positive (eg, social support, self-expression) than parents who were more likely to view social media engagement as either being inconsequential (eg, something to do when teens are bored) or interfering with completing necessary activities and tasks.[77] This highlights the potential discrepancy between youth and parents in how they understand and approach the function of technology in the lives of youth.

Given the necessity of using technology to adjust to COVID-19 restrictions, technology use and screen time soared among youth during the pandemic. Reports indicate that screen time has more than doubled among youth during the pandemic and that this impacted even our youngest children with a sample of kindergarten students averaging 6.6 hours of media use a day, with weekday use exceeding weekend use (6.8 hours and 5.8 hours, respectively).[78] Of note, all aspects of technology use, with the exception of connecting via video, was highest among parents and children, with higher rates of anxiety underscoring the complicated interplay and unknown directionality between technology use and anxiety.[76] Furthermore, the impact of prolonged screen time on youth's mental health remains to be validated. However, it is likely that a subset of youth has developed PIU and will have difficulty transitioning back to use patterns that were more common before the pandemic. It will also be necessary for organizations to re-examine screen time guidelines and to provide ongoing guidance to practitioners and parents for ways to support youth's engagement with technology and social media in a postpandemic world.

As pandemic guidelines and restrictions change, it is important for clinicians to be aware of ways to support youth through these transitions. It is likely that a large portion of youth will experience residual distress and negative mental health outcomes due to the large-scale and long-standing nature of the COVID-19 pandemic.[73] Clinicians should routinely screen for anxiety and trauma symptoms in both children and parents and subsequently refer these families to relevant mental health services. Clinicians should also assess trends in technology usage of their patients and caregivers over the course of the pandemic to facilitate the development of a media transition plan that can help families balance the time spent online and offline. Finally, clinicians could support the development of guidelines and agreements between adolescents and parents; one that focuses on balancing the need for adolescent autonomy with parent's desire to have appropriate protections in place for online use.[77]

WHERE DO WE POKÉMON GO FROM HERE: VENTURING INTO THE WORLD

When the original article was published in 2018,[79] a description of the phenomenon of Pokémon Go, an augmented reality (AR) smartphone game introduced in the summer of 2016, was included. People of all ages rapidly embraced this game, which was played by an estimated 44 million people worldwide at the height of its popularity.[80,81] Pokémon Go encouraged exploration and activity by requiring players to physically travel around their communities seeking virtual treasures.[82] Anecdotally, child mental health providers have described children with severe social phobia, separation anxiety, and agoraphobia who were motivated to leave home to play Pokémon Go. Additional research examining the role of AR games among children in teens is needed, but these results suggest that AR games may prove useful in encouraging physical activity and social engagement and could serve to reduce symptoms of anxiety.[80–82] As our world opens after the pandemic, new AR platforms may be necessary to support the exposure for the socially anxious to leave the home.

SUMMARY
Recommendations for Providers

Despite limitations, current research related to online habits and anxiety reveals important considerations for mental health providers. Clinicians should assess online activity beyond simply assessing total time spent online, including specific aspects of use and individual factors that inform associated risks. The following points provide guidance for providers gathering information about the internet habits of young patients during clinical interviews:

- Type and frequency of online activities: What are the primary online activities (eg, YouTube, instant messaging [IM], social media, gaming) and how much time is spent on each? What is the general content, and does it include age-inappropriate material or interactions? How many social media accounts are currently being used?

- Active versus passive use: How much time online is spent actively posting content (text, pictures, videos) or engaged in real-time communication (IM, chatrooms)? How much time online is spent passively viewing content?
- Emotional valence: Is the content viewed and shared primarily positive (liking others' posts, communicating positive messages or stories about one's own life) or negative (unhappy status updates, sharing frustrations, critical or contentious interactions with others)?
- Beliefs and attitudes: Do individuals prefer online communication over face-to-face interactions? If so, why? How important are either the need for social assurance or FOMO as motivators for online engagement?
- What is the balance of screen time use, physical activity, and restful sleep? What times of day are screens being used, and how is screen time impacting sleep habits, quantity, and quality?
- Positive or avoidant coping skills: Is the youth using online activity to extend real-life friendships or spending time online avoiding school and other interpersonal interactions?
- Virtual gaming: Does the patient meet criteria for internet or video game addiction? If so, providers need to prioritize treatment of IVGA because these patterns have been found to predict the subsequent development of anxiety disorders.[37]

Technology is rapidly changing and will continue to come with both opportunities and hazards. Therefore, it is important for mental health providers to understand that virtual platforms including the internet and social media play an important role in the social development of young patients and to advise patients and families how online habits can either exacerbate or alleviate anxiety. Online resources (see **Table 2**) are also available to support parents to guide children and teens in traversing the virtual world.

A NEW NORMAL?

This original article was revised between April and June 2021, at a time when vaccines were offered for children aged 12 years and older, and hope was being held for "herd immunity" to the COVID-19 virus. However, the pandemic occurred at a time with rapid opportunities and changes to virtual technology platforms. Social distancing and lockdowns led to greatly increased screen time, less in-person socialization, less physical activity, and time in nonvirtual technology play. Time online allowed friendships to be developed and to continue, creativity emerged for live stream, peer-to-peer physical activities leading to decreased childhood anxiety,[83] and it is unclear what the "new normal" will be with respect to youth and virtual technology. Stay tuned…

CLINICS CARE POINTS

- Problematic Internet Use is a condition where youth experience obsessive thoughts about being online, have difficulty unplugging from devices, and experience disruptions in activities of daily living due to excessive time spent online.
- Clinicians working with youth need to routinely assess technology use including frequency, duration, quality of content, and impact of use on adaptive skills. Social networks can provide an important source of support and networking for youth who are members of marginalized groups (e.g. LGBTQPIA).
- There is a large research to practice gap for electronic and mobile health interventions, especially mental health apps for youth, so clinicians need to help support families in understanding how to evaluate and utilize these technologies.

> • The COVID-19 pandemic resulted in youth across ages engaging in far more screen time than previously recommended and researchers are now re-evaluating the effectiveness of screen time as a guideline versus shifting to a focus of ensuring that technology is not interfering with sleep, physical activities, school work, and interpersonal relationships.

ACKNOWLEDGMENTS

The authors thank Paul Weigle, MD, and Kristopher Kaliebe, MD, for the original invitation to participate in the 2018 *Child and Adolescent Psychiatric Clinics of NA: Youth Internet Habits & Mental Health*.

DISCLOSURE

The authors have nothing to disclose.

REFERENCES

1. Angold A, Costello EJ, Erkanli A. Comorbidity. J Child Psychol Psychiatry 1999; 40(1):57–87.
2. Kessler RC, Berglund P, Demler O, et al. Lifetime prevalence and age-of-onset distributions of DSM-IV disorders in the national comorbidity survey replication. Arch Gen Psychiatry 2005;62(6):593–602.
3. Hawes MT, Szenczy AK, Klein DN, et al. Increases in depression and anxiety symptoms in adolescents and young adults during the covid-19 pandemic. Psychol Med 2021;1–9. https://doi.org/10.1017/s0033291720005358.
4. Courtney D, Watson P, Battaglia M, et al. Covid-19 impacts on child and youth anxiety and depression: challenges and opportunities. Can J Psychiatry 2020; 65(10):688–91.
5. Deolmi M, Pisani F. Psychological and psychiatric impact of covid-19 pandemic among children and adolescents. Acta Biomed 2020;91(4):e2020149.
6. #statusofmind social media and young people's mental health and wellbeing. 2017. Available at: https://www.rsph.org.uk/static/uploaded/d125b27c-0b62-41c5-a2c0155a8887cd01.pdf. Accessed June 1, 2021.
7. Oberst U, Wegmann E, Stodt B, et al. Negative consequences from heavy social networking in adolescents: the mediating role of fear of missing out. J Adolesc 2017;55:51–60.
8. Domingues-Montanari S. Clinical and psychological effects of excessive screen time on children. J Paediatr Child Health 2017;53(4):333–8.
9. Hoge E, Bickham D, Cantor J. Digital media, anxiety, and depression in children. Pediatrics 2017;140(Suppl 2):S76–80.
10. Muzaffar N, Brito EB, Fogel J, et al. The association of adolescent facebook behaviours with symptoms of social anxiety, generalized anxiety, and depression. J Can Acad Child Adolesc Psychiatry 2018;27(4):252–60.
11. Ohannessian CM. Video game play and anxiety during late adolescence: the moderating effects of gender and social context. J Affect Disord 2018;226:216–9.
12. Zink J, Belcher BR, Imm K, et al. The relationship between screen-based sedentary behaviors and symptoms of depression and anxiety in youth: a systematic review of moderating variables. BMC Public Health 2020;20(1):472.
13. Bauman S, Rivers I. Virtual worlds. Mental health in the digital age. London: Palgrave Macmillan UK; 2015. p. 117–40.

14. Adıbelli D, Sümen A. The effect of the coronavirus (covid-19) pandemic on health-related quality of life in children. Child Youth Serv Rev 2020;119:105595.
15. Common sense media: age-based media reviews for families. 2021. Available at: https://www.commonsensemedia.org. [Accessed 8 June 2021].
16. US states oppose a children's version of instagram. AFP News, International Business Times; 2021. Available at: https://www.ibtimes.com/us-states-oppose-childrens-version-instagram-3196298. [Accessed 17 May 2021].
17. Zolyomi A, Schmalz M. Mining for social skills: minecraft in home and therapy for neurodiverse youth. In: Proceedings of the 50th Hawaii International Conference on System Sciences. 2017. https://doi.org/10.24251/HICSS.2017.411.
18. Taheri E, Heshmat R, Esmaeil Motlagh M, et al. Association of physical activity and screen time with psychiatric distress in children and adolescents: CASPIAN-IV study. J Trop Pediatr 2019;65(4):361–72.
19. Thorisdottir IE, Sigurvinsdottir R, Kristjansson AL, et al. Longitudinal association between social media use and psychological distress among adolescents. Prev Med 2020;141:106270.
20. Twenge JM, Hisler GC, Krizan Z. Associations between screen time and sleep duration are primarily driven by portable electronic devices: evidence from a population-based study of U.S. children ages 0-17. Sleep Med 2019;56:211–8.
21. Valkenburg PM, Peter J. Online communication among adolescents: an integrated model of its attraction, opportunities, and risks. J Adolesc Health 2011;48(2):121–7.
22. Caplan SE. Relations among loneliness, social anxiety, and problematic internet use. Cyberpsychol Behav 2007;10(2):234–42.
23. Prizant-Passal S, Shechner T, Aderka IM. Social anxiety and internet use–a meta-analysis: what do we know? What are we missing? Comput Human Behav 2016;62:221–9.
24. Rauch SM, Strobel C, Bella M, et al. Face to face versus facebook: does exposure to social networking web sites augment or attenuate physiological arousal among the socially anxious? Cyberpsychol Behav Soc Netw 2014;17(3):187–90.
25. Choukas-Bradley S, Nesi J, Widman L, et al. The appearance-related social media consciousness scale: development and validation with adolescents. Body Image 2020;33:164–74.
26. Sharma M, Amandeep, Mathur DM, et al. Nomophobia and its relationship with depression, anxiety, and quality of life in adolescents. Ind Psychiatry J 2019;28(2):231–6.
27. Xie X, Xie J. Parental phubbing accelerates depression in late childhood and adolescence: a two-path model. J Adolesc 2020;78:43–52.
28. Ergun G, Alkan A. The social media disorder and ostracism in adolescents: (ostraca- sm study). Eurasian J Med 2020;52(2):139–44.
29. Khalil SA, Kamal H, Elkholy H. The prevalence of problematic internet use among a sample of egyptian adolescents and its psychiatric comorbidities. Int J Soc Psychiatry 2020. https://doi.org/10.1177/0020764020983841. 20764020983841.
30. Throuvala MA, Griffiths MD, Rennoldson M, et al. Perceived challenges and online harms from social media use on a severity continuum: a qualitative psychological stakeholder perspective. Int J Environ Res Public Health 2021;18(6):3227.
31. Zdanowicz N, Reynaert C, Jacques D, et al. Screen time and (belgian) teenagers. Psychiatr Danub 2020;32(Suppl 1):36–41.
32. Lee-Won RJ, Herzog L, Park SG. Hooked on facebook: the role of social anxiety and need for social assurance in problematic use of facebook. Cyberpsychol Behav Soc Netw 2015;18(10):567–74.

33. Wood MA, Bukowski WM, Lis E. The digital self: how social media serves as a setting that shapes youth's emotional experiences. Adolesc Res Rev 2016;1(2): 163–73.

34. Charmaraman L, Richer AM, Liu C, et al. Early adolescent social media-related body dissatisfaction: associations with depressive symptoms, social anxiety, peers, and celebrities. J Dev Behav Pediatr 2021. https://doi.org/10.1097/DBP.0000000000000911.

35. Ohannessian CM, Fagle T, Salafia C. Social media use and internalizing symptoms during early adolescence: the role of co-rumination. J Affect Disord 2021; 280(Pt A):85–8. https://doi.org/10.1016/j.jad.2020.10.079.

36. Kim S, Favotto L, Halladay J, et al. Differential associations between passive and active forms of screen time and adolescent mood and anxiety disorders. Soc Psychiatry Psychiatr Epidemiol 2020;55(11):1469–78.

37. Gentile DA, Choo H, Liau A, et al. Pathological video game use among youths: a two-year longitudinal study. Pediatrics 2011;127(2):e319–29.

38. Primack BA, Escobar-Viera CG. Social media as it interfaces with psychosocial development and mental illness in transitional age youth. Child Adolesc Psychiatr Clin N Am 2017;26(2):217–33.

39. Byron P, Albury K, Evers C. "It would be weird to have that on facebook": young people's use of social media and the risk of sharing sexual health information. Reprod Health Matters 2013;21(41):35–44.

40. Chou H-TG, Edge N. "They are happier and having better lives than i am": the impact of using facebook on perceptions of others' lives. Cyberpsychol Behav Soc Netw 2012;15(2):117–21.

41. Laghi F, Schneider BH, Vitoroulis I, et al. Knowing when not to use the internet: shyness and adolescents' on-line and off-line interactions with friends. Comput Human Behav 2013;29(1):51–7.

42. Vannucci A, Flannery KM, Ohannessian CM. Social media use and anxiety in emerging adults. J Affect Disord 2017;207:163–6.

43. Selkie E, Adkins V, Masters E, et al. Transgender adolescents' uses of social media for social support. J Adolesc Health 2020;66(3):275–80.

44. Nolan S, Hendricks J, Towell A. Adolescent mothers' use of social networking sites creating positive mental health outcomes. Aust Nurs Midwifery J 2016; 23(11):50.

45. Odgers CL, Jensen MR. Annual research review: adolescent mental health in the digital age: Facts, fears, and future directions. J Child Psychol Psychiatry 2020; 61(3):336–48.

46. Chaudron S. Young children (0-8) and digital technology a qualitative exploratory study across seven countries. Luxembourg: Publications Office; 2016.

47. O'Keeffe GS, Clarke-Pearson K. The impact of social media on children, adolescents, and families. Pediatrics 2011;127(4):800–4.

48. Hadjipanayis A, Efstathiou E, Altorjai P, et al. Social media and children: what is the paediatrician's role? Eur J Pediatr 2019;178(10):1605–12.

49. Park S, Chang HY, Park EJ, et al. Maternal depression and children's screen overuse. J Korean Med Sci 2018;33(34):e219.

50. Ruggieri S, Santoro G, Pace U, et al. Problematic facebook use and anxiety concerning use of social media in mothers and their offspring: an actor-partner interdependence model. Addict Behav Rep 2020;11:100256.

51. Solecki S. The smart use of smartphones in pediatrics. J Pediatr Nurs 2020; 55:6–9.

52. Stiglic N, Viner RM. Effects of screentime on the health and well-being of children and adolescents: a systematic review of reviews. BMJ Open 2019;9(1):e023191.
53. Radovic A, Gmelin T, Stein B, et al. Depressed adolescents' positive and negative use of social media. J Adolesc 2017;55:5–15.
54. Lindhiem O, Bennett CB, Rosen D, et al. Mobile technology boosts the effectiveness of psychotherapy and behavioral interventions: a meta-analysis. Behav Modif 2015;39(6):785–804.
55. Morgan AJ, Rapee RM, Salim A, et al. Internet-delivered parenting program for prevention and early intervention of anxiety problems in young children: randomized controlled trial. J Am Acad Child Adolesc Psychiatry 2017;56(5):417–25.e1.
56. Archangeli C, Marti FA, Wobga-Pasiah EA, et al. Mobile health interventions for psychiatric conditions in children: a scoping review: a scoping review. Child Adolesc Psychiatr Clin N Am 2017;26(1):13–31.
57. Whiteside SP. Mobile device-based applications for childhood anxiety disorders. J Child Adolesc Psychopharmacol 2016;26(3):246–51.
58. Bry LJ, Chou T, Miguel E, et al. Consumer smartphone apps marketed for child and adolescent anxiety: a systematic review and content analysis. Behav Ther 2018;49(2):249–61.
59. Stoll RD, Pina AA, Gary K, et al. Usability of a smartphone application to support the prevention and early intervention of anxiety in youth. Cogn Behav Pract 2017. https://doi.org/10.1016/j.cbpra.2016.11.002.
60. Grist R, Porter J, Stallard P. Mental health mobile apps for preadolescents and adolescents: a systematic review. J Med Internet Res 2017;19(5):e176.
61. Qu C, Sas C, Dauden Roquet C, et al. Functionality of top-rated mobile apps for depression: systematic search and evaluation. JMIR Ment Health 2020;7(1): e15321.
62. Ridout B, Campbell A. The use of social networking sites in mental health interventions for young people: systematic review. J Med Internet Res 2018;20(12): e12244.
63. App advisor: an american psychiatry association initiative. American Psychiatric Association (APA). Available at: https://www.psychiatry.org/psychiatrists/practice/mental-health-apps. Accessed May 17, 2021.
64. Christensen H, Batterham P, Calear A. Online interventions for anxiety disorders. Curr Opin Psychiatry 2014;27(1):7–13.
65. Nordh M, Wahlund T, Jolstedt M, et al. Therapist-guided internet-delivered cognitive behavioral therapy vs internet-delivered supportive therapy for children and adolescents with social anxiety disorder: a randomized clinical trial. JAMA Psychiatry 2021. https://doi.org/10.1001/jamapsychiatry.2021.0469.
66. Aspvall K, Andersson E, Melin K, et al. Effect of an internet-delivered stepped-care program vs in-person cognitive behavioral therapy on obsessive-compulsive disorder symptoms in children and adolescents: a randomized clinical trial. JAMA 2021;325(18):1863–73.
67. Patel A, Schieble T, Davidson M, et al. Distraction with a hand-held video game reduces pediatric preoperative anxiety. Paediatric Anaesth 2006;16(10):1019–27.
68. Seiden SC, McMullan S, Sequera-Ramos L, et al. Tablet-based interactive distraction (tbid) vs oral midazolam to minimize perioperative anxiety in pediatric patients: a noninferiority randomized trial. Paediatric Anaesth 2014;24(12): 1217–23.
69. Thabrew H, Stasiak K, Garcia-Hoyos V, et al. Game for health: how ehealth approaches might address the psychological needs of children and young people with long-term physical conditions. J Paediatr Child Health 2016;52(11):1012–8.

70. Wiederhold MD, Gao K, Wiederhold BK. Clinical use of virtual reality distraction system to reduce anxiety and pain in dental procedures. Cyberpsychol Behav Soc Netw 2014;17(6):359–65.

71. McGar AB, Kindler C, Marsac M. Electronic health interventions for preventing and treating negative psychological sequelae resulting from pediatric medical conditions: systematic review. JMIR Pediatr Parent 2019;2(2):e12427.

72. Francisco R, Pedro M, Delvecchio E, et al. Psychological symptoms and behavioral changes in children and adolescents during the early phase of covid-19 quarantine in three european countries. Front Psychiatry 2020;11:570164.

73. Imran N, Aamer I, Sharif MI, et al. Psychological burden of quarantine in children and adolescents: a rapid systematic review and proposed solutions. Pak J Med Sci 2020;36(5):1106–16.

74. Alves JM, Yunker AG, DeFendis A, et al. Associations between affect, physical activity, and anxiety among us children during covid-19. medRxiv 2020. https://doi.org/10.1101/2020.10.20.20216424.

75. Guessoum SB, Lachal J, Radjack R, et al. Adolescent psychiatric disorders during the covid-19 pandemic and lockdown. Psychiatry Res 2020;291:113264.

76. Drouin M, McDaniel BT, Pater J, et al. How parents and their children used social media and technology at the beginning of the covid-19 pandemic and associations with anxiety. Cyberpsychol Behav Soc Netw 2020;23(11):727–36.

77. Biernesser C, Montano G, Miller E, et al. Social media use and monitoring for adolescents with depression and implications for the covid-19 pandemic: qualitative study of parent and child perspectives. JMIR Pediatr Parent 2020;3(2):e21644.

78. Dore RA, Purtell KM, Justice LM. Media use among kindergarteners from low-income households during the covid-19 shutdown. J Dev Behav Pediatr 2021. https://doi.org/10.1097/dbp.0000000000000955.

79. Glover J, Fritsch SL. #kidsanxiety and social media: a review. Child Adolesc Psychiatr Clin N Am 2018;27(2):171–82.

80. Bonus JA, Peebles A, Mares M-L, et al. Look on the bright side (of media effects): Pokémon go as a catalyst for positive life experiences. Media Psychology 2017;21(2):263–87.

81. Dotinga R. Gotta catch 'em all: is pokémon go an intervention for schizophrenia? Clinical Psychiatry News Blog 2017. Available at: http://www.mdedge.com/clinicalpsychiatrynews/article/135375/schizophrenia-other-psychotic-disorders/gotta-catch-em-all. [Accessed 4 July 2017].

82. Howe KB, Suharlim C, Ueda P, et al. Gotta catch'em all! Pokémon go and physical activity among young adults: difference in differences study. BMJ 2016;355:i6270.

83. Zheng Y, Wang W, Zhong Y, et al. A peer-to-peer live-streaming intervention for children during covid-19 homeschooling to promote physical activity and reduce anxiety and eye strain: cluster randomized controlled trial. J Med Internet Res 2021;23(4):e24316.

Childhood Trauma and Psychosis

A Brief Updated Review and Case Study

Yael Dvir, MD

KEYWORDS

- Childhood trauma • Psychosis • Psychotic illness
- Posttraumatic stress disorder (PTSD)
- PTSD with secondary psychotic features (PTSD-SPs) • Ultra–high-risk (UHR)
- Transition to psychosis (TTP) • First-episode psychosis (FEP)

KEY POINTS

- Childhood trauma and psychosis are linked, such that childhood trauma is a significant risk factor for psychosis.
- Childhood trauma is associated with a more severe presentation of psychotic illness with a dose-response effect.
- Evidence suggests that patients at ultra--high risk (UHR) for psychosis experienced higher rates of exposure to childhood trauma (54%–90%) and exposure to more severe trauma and that childhood trauma is associated with UHR transition to psychosis.
- In individuals with psychotic illness, childhood trauma doubles the risk of violent behavior.
- Acceptance and commitment therapy for psychosis and trauma is a promising psychotherapeutic intervention for this population.

INTRODUCTION

The author's reviews in *Child and Adolescent Psychiatric Clinics of North America*, from 2013 and 2020, concluded that childhood trauma and psychosis are linked, such that childhood trauma is a significant risk factor for psychosis.[1,2] This is evident in studies showing higher rates of psychotic symptoms in children with trauma histories, and higher rates of childhood trauma in first-episode psychosis (FEP) patients. A large longitudinal population-based study showed that in youth who experienced childhood trauma in the first 17 years of life, the risk for experiencing psychotic symptoms was 2.5 times to 2.9 times higher compared with those who did not experience such events, and 4.7 times to 5 times higher for those who experienced 3 or more such events.[3] In addition, childhood trauma is associated with a more severe presentation of psychotic

Department of Psychiatry, University of Massachusetts Chan Medical School, 55 Lake Avenue North, Worcester, MA 01655, USA
E-mail address: Yael.Dvir@umassmed.edu

Child Adolesc Psychiatric Clin N Am 31 (2022) 91–98
https://doi.org/10.1016/j.chc.2021.08.002
1056-4993/22/© 2021 Elsevier Inc. All rights reserved.

childpsych.theclinics.com

illness: perceptual disturbance, affective instability, suicidality, and substance use all are heightened. There also is a clear dose-response effect: increased severity of positive psychotic symptoms is associated with higher numbers of traumatic events, whereas negative symptom severity is associated with childhood neglect.[1,2]

This clinical update sheds light on aspects that were less emphasized in the earlier summaries. It begins with a case illustrating these points and discusses the relationship between mood, anxiety, posttraumatic stress disorder (PTSD), and psychosis. Then, childhood trauma and the ultra–high risk (UHR) for psychosis state and the relationship between childhood adversity and trauma and violence toward others in individuals with psychosis are discussed and several innovative psychotherapeutic treatment approaches described.

CASE STUDY: PRIMARY PSYCHOTIC ILLNESS TRIGGERED BY TRAUMA OR POSTTRAUMATIC STRESS DISORDER WITH SECONDARY PSYCHOSIS?
Case Presentation

K is a 17-year-old adolescent boy who was referred to the author by his treating child and adolescent psychiatrist for consultation, to aid with diagnostic clarification in a youth with significant mood symptoms, PTSD diagnosis, and persistent and distressing symptoms of psychosis that have not responded to several trials of antipsychotic medications. K reported that medications have not been helpful, and that psychotherapy has been "superficially helpful." He reported that for the past 2 years he has experienced auditory hallucinations of 10 different voices and visual hallucinations of bugs and figures that are distracting and scary to him. He also reported feeling as if he is watched and in the past 6 months that others are putting thoughts into his head or that he is thinking thoughts that are not his own. He reported feeling "a bit depressed," numb, and lacking emotions. He first struggled with depression 3 years ago (and had met diagnostic criteria for a major depressive episode). K identified exposure to a sibling's severe behavioral dysregulation within the home as a traumatizing event. K described himself as a shy and somewhat anxious young child and added that he has many missing pieces and lost memories from his earlier childhood. He reported that he is a good student but recently has been struggling with school attendance and feeling overwhelmed by schoolwork. He has close friendships, which he continues to maintain. When specifically asked, K reported that the content of the voices was self-derogatory, telling him he is "not good enough." His difficulties with school attendance appeared connected to social anxiety. K was articulate, well groomed, and friendly. His thought process was organized. His affect was constricted and at times he appeared detached from the described experiences. In a separate interview, his mother described additional stressors within the home, including the father's alcohol use and resulting emotional dysregulation and K witnessing 2 suicide attempts by his mother. She also reported that K's depression has not abated in the past 3 years and that he has never experienced psychotic symptoms independent of mood symptoms.

Clinical Questions

Given the severity of K's psychotic symptoms, which include multiple voices, paranoid ideations, and thought insertion, is K suffering from early-onset schizophrenia or schizoaffective disorder? How should his treatment team approach his care?

DISCUSSION

K presented with a developmental history consistent of shy temperament and social anxiety and significant interpersonal traumatic experiences within the home throughout his childhood. He has experienced mood symptoms consistent with major depressive disorder and experienced psychotic symptoms, most of which are congruent with his mood state. He has not had any cognitive or social functional deterioration. He also exhibited symptoms of PTSD, including distress when with his sibling, negative thoughts and affect, hypervigilance, and difficulty concentrating. Therefore, the diagnostic formulation concluded that K can best be described as experiencing co-occurring major depressive disorder with psychotic features and PTSD. Alternatively, a diagnosis of PTSD with secondary psychotic features (PTSD-SPs) was discussed with the family.

Childhood trauma has varied consequences, with most individuals never developing psychiatric sequela, and those who do develop a variety of psychiatric disorders, including anxiety, mood, psychotic disorders, and PTSD. There is an overlap between symptoms of PTSD and psychosis, making this distinction especially challenging for treating clinicians; there also is emerging evidence that PTSD-SP may be an independent subtype of PTSD with its distinct features and risk factors.[4] As is illustrated in this case, PTSD-SPs tends to present as PTSD with positive psychotic symptoms, some (but not all) related to the trauma experience but no significant thought disorder. This case demonstrates the importance of examining the contributions of mood and anxiety symptoms to the relationship between childhood trauma and psychosis. Psychosis in youth continues to be most seen commonly in the context of mood disorders.[5] In addition, there is support for mood, anxiety, and PTSD as mediating factors, suggesting "affective pathways to psychosis."[6] Repeated traumas may have a cumulative effect on emotional regulation, linking the relationship between the number of traumas and their severity and the risk of developing of psychosis. Furthermore, childhood trauma that occurs within the context of interpersonal relationships with caretakers and in the context of attachment may result in difficulty trusting others, worries about relationships, and social withdrawal.[7]

CHILDHOOD TRAUMA, BORDERLINE PERSONALITY DISORDER, AND PSYCHOTIC SYMPTOMS

Childhood trauma also is considered an etiologic factor contributing to the development of borderline personality disorder, especially when considered as part of a multifactorial model.[8] In addition, the diagnostic criteria for borderline personality disorder include periods of stress-related paranoia and loss of contact with reality, lasting from a few minutes to a few hours, which can be distressing. Additionally, patients with borderline personality disorder have high rates of co-occurring mood disorders.[9] Baryshnikov and colleagues (2018)[10] examined wherever features of borderline personality disorders in patients with mood disorders may help explain the relationship between childhood trauma and psychotic experiences in those patients, specifically severe dissociation and transient paranoid ideations, and found that cognitive and perceptual symptoms appear to mediate this relationship.

CHILDHOOD TRAUMA AND ULTRA-HIGH RISK FOR PSYCHOSIS

UHR is a term describing individuals at high risk for developing psychosis and is internationally defined as attenuated psychotic symptoms (onset/worsening of subthreshold psychosis in the past 12 months), brief and limited psychotic symptoms (onset of transient psychotic symptoms for less than 1 week), and genetic risk and deterioration syndrome (schizotypal personality disorder or first-degree relative with psychotic illness, with decreased function in past year). Its importance is recognized for the purpose of identifying individuals who may benefit from early psychosis intervention. In a meta-analysis from 2017, Fusar-Poli and colleagues[11] examined environmental risk factors for psychosis in those with UHR for psychosis by reviewing 44 studies that included 54 risk factors. They concluded that the risk of UHR transition to psychosis (TTP) is significantly higher than that of the general population, reaching 29% at 2 years, after which it plateaus and reaches 35% after 10 years. The relative risk for developing psychosis at 2 years is 460, compared with the general population, but there does not appear to be a higher risk for developing other psychiatric illness. Obstetric complications were a significantly associated prenatal/perinatal complication, and there was strong evidence that childhood trauma, childhood emotional abuse, childhood physical neglect, and high perceived stress were associated with UHR TTP.[11] This is important because a better understanding of how childhood trauma contributes to UHR, and more specifically to UHR TTP, will help improve prediction and early intervention in this population.

Another systematic review assessed the severity and prevalence of childhood adversities, defined as exposure to childhood trauma and bullying and/or victimization in individuals with UHR and examined their correlations with UHR TTP. Peh and colleagues (2019)[12] reported that UHR participants experienced higher rates of exposure to childhood trauma (54%–90%) and exposure to more severe trauma. Because the studies reviewed used different trauma assessments, which defined trauma subtypes differently, there was high heterogenicity within abuse subtypes. Bullying and victimization experiences, however, were reported 3.9 times more frequently in the UHR participants compared with healthy controls, ranging from 33.3% to 66.7% across the 3 countries in which these studies were conducted. The investigators also examined wherever there was an association between childhood adversity, UHR, and TTP and did not find one; however, they did find a link between childhood sexual trauma and TTP.[12]

CHILDHOOD ADVERSITY AND VIOLENCE TO OTHERS IN INDIVIDUALS WITH PSYCHOSIS

Acknowledging that the relationship between childhood trauma and psychosis in adults is supported by significant evidence, Green and colleagues (2019)[13] explored the impact of this relationship on risk to violence toward others. They analyzed 11 cross-sectional or case-control design studies (N = 2215), showing that in individuals with psychotic illness, childhood trauma doubles the risk of violent behavior. Experiencing violence in childhood has been identified as a risk factor for being a victim of and perpetrating reactive violence in adulthood, whereas witnessing domestic violence in childhood is a risk factor for perpetrating intimate partner violence. There also may be a relationship between symptom acuity, severity, and violent content of hallucinations and risk of violence toward other. As such, childhood trauma, which increases psychotic illness acuity and severity, may be associated with increased risk of violence toward others. The investigators also note that all the studies included in their analysis have participants with psychotic illness who experienced childhood trauma and have never been violent, so that studying protective factors in order to implement preventative strategies is a critically important next step.[13]

ADVANCES IN PSYCHOTHERAPEUTIC APPROACHES IN THE TREATMENT OF TRAUMA AND PSYCHOSIS

Cognitive therapy for command hallucinations (CTCH) is a targeted cognitive-behavior therapy (CBT) offering up to 25 sessions administered up to 9 months, designed to assist patients who experience such symptoms decrease their responses to commands and therefore reduce distress and unwanted behaviors. At 18 months, participants who received CTCH were less likely to experience recurrence of "harmful compliance" (28%) compared with the control group (45%), accompanied by a reduction in their beliefs about power of the voices. The researchers defined "cognitive affective dimension of voice hearing" as measures of beliefs about voices power and threat, childhood trauma, depression, and self-harm and found that it strongly predicted harmful compliance to command hallucinations at 18 months from treatment initiation.[14]

ACCEPTANCE AND COMMITMENT THERAPY FOR PSYCHOSIS AND TRAUMA

Acceptance and commitment therapy (ACT) is an empirically based method of psychotherapy that uses cognitive-behavior principles, acceptance, commitment, and mindfulness strategies. It has been studied separately as a treatment of psychosis and for trauma-related sequela.[15] Spidel and colleagues[15] evaluated its effectiveness for treating patients who have both a psychotic illness and history of childhood trauma. Given that low treatment adherence and engagement with service has been shown to be correlated with both psychotic illness and childhood trauma, they chose to evaluate effectiveness of ACT on treatment compliance. Similarly, because childhood trauma has been shown to cause significant emotional dysregulation as part of many possible sequela, which in turn has been correlated with more severe symptom distress,[16] the investigators also evaluated ACTs effect on emotional regulation and symptom distress. This study used a modified group-based ACT intervention for participants with psychosis and trauma histories, which included mindfulness meditation (shown beneficial to individuals with early psychosis) and spanned 10 sessions so that relevant skills were covered more comprehensively; 50 participants ranging in age from 19 years to 64 years were randomized into ACT and treatment and usual groups. The ACT group participants had an increase in emotion regulation and acceptance as measured by the acceptance scale Cognitive Emotion Regulation Questionnaire, decrease in symptom severity as measured by the Brief Psychiatric Rating Scale and Generalized Anxiety Disorder scale, and improved engagement in treatment (especially help seeking) immediately after treatment and at 3 months following its completion. Contrary to other ACT protocols, which focused on trauma alone, participants did not experience a significant reduction in trauma symptoms in this study. This can be explained by the short duration of the intervention.[15] In a follow-up study, Spidel and colleagues (2019)[17] examined predictors of outcome for ACT for psychosis and trauma, which included trauma severity, age, attachment, mindfulness, and number of sessions attended. Given that frequency and severity of childhood trauma have been shown predictors of psychosis and emotional dysregulation severity, they are important considerations when evaluating treatment effectiveness. The investigators found that severity of childhood trauma did not cause a lesser response to ACT and that participants with higher severity rates of childhood trauma had similar response compared with those with lesser severity, suggesting that ACT may be a suitable treatment of individuals with psychosis and trauma regardless of childhood trauma severity.[17]

EVIDENCE-BASED INTERVENTIONS FOR POSTTRAUMATIC STRESS DISORDER IN FIRST-EPISODE PSYCHOSIS

There is limited evidence to guide psychotherapeutic interventions in young people with FEP and co-occurring PTSD. Much of this is because of clinicians' reluctance to use trauma-specific interventions in this patient population, because of concerns that this may result in symptom exacerbation and destabilization. Additionally, psychosis often is an exclusion criterion from studies examining trauma-focused psychotherapies. This is important because childhood trauma is highly prevalent among individuals with FEP, as is co-occurring PTSD. There is ample evidence to suggest that trauma-focused psychotherapy is effective and safe for PTSD and that, although a minority of those who undergo trauma-focused psychotherapy report initial symptom exacerbation with later improvement, those on waitlists show more exacerbation, suggestion that no treatment is more harmful.[18] Tong and colleagues (2017)[18] sought to better understand participants' reactions to a treatment that included distress management, assessment of trauma and trauma-related symptoms, trauma-related patient education, and trauma-based formulation by conducting semistructured interviews with 8 patients with FEP and PTSD participating in this intervention. Participants' responses were varied, and. although all participants reported that the intervention was beneficial and worthwhile and that they would recommend it to others in their situation, all but 1 participant reported distress in sessions where they discussed their trauma, and half reported distress and symptom exacerbation (including psychotic symptoms) outside of sessions. The investigators concluded that distress and symptom increase do not indicate that participants with FEP are not responding to the trauma-focused psychotherapeutic intervention.[18] These are important factors to consider, however, when offering informed consent and support throughout this intervention.

SUMMARY

Significant evidence suggests strong links between childhood trauma and psychosis, with childhood trauma considered a significant risk factor for psychosis, causing a more severe presentation of psychotic illness with a dose-response effect. Additionally, the relationship between anxiety, mood, PTSD, borderline personality disorder, and childhood trauma and psychosis and the difficulties distinguishing between overlapping symptoms require careful attention of the treating clinician considering the presentation and treatment course. This is true for young people with UHR and FEP. There also appears to be a link between childhood trauma and violent behavior in individuals with psychotic illness. Finally, more research is needed into the effectiveness and safety of trauma-focused psychotherapeutic interventions, but ACT for psychosis and trauma appears to have beneficial impact, and other interventions with emphasis on CBT approaches and psychoeducation appear effective and safe even when temporary distress and symptom exacerbation are reported.

CLINICS CARE POINTS

- When assessing patients with childhood trauma and psychotic symptoms, the clinician should note overlapping presentations of PTSD and psychosis, because this is critical when differentiating between PTSD, PTSD-SPs, mood disorder with psychotic symptoms, and primary psychotic illness.

- When assessing patients with UHR or FEP, careful consideration should be given to obtaining childhood trauma history, which can be an important prognostic factor with significant importance when implementing psychotherapeutic interventions.

- Although symptom exacerbation remains a concern when implementing trauma-focused psychotherapy in patients with childhood trauma and psychotic illness, emerging evidence suggests that under careful clinical care those interventions overall are beneficial and well received by patients.

DISCLOSURE

The author has nothing to disclose.

REFERENCES

1. Stanton KJ, Denietolis B, Goodwin BJ, et al. Childhood trauma and psychosis: an updated review. Child Adolesc Psychiatr Clin N Am 2020;29(1):115–29.
2. Dvir Y, Denietolis B, Frazier JA. Childhood trauma and psychosis. Child Adolesc Psychiatr Clin N Am 2013;22(4):629–41.
3. Croft J, Heron J, Teufel C, et al. Association of trauma type, age of exposure, and frequency in childhood and adolescence with psychotic experiences in early adulthood. JAMA Psychiatry 2019;76(1):79–86.
4. Compean E, Hamner M. Posttraumatic stress disorder with secondary psychotic features (PTSD-SP): diagnostic and treatment challenges. Prog Neuropsychopharmacol Biol Psychiatry 2019;88:265–75.
5. Carlson GA. Affective disorders and psychosis in youth. Child Adolesc Psychiatr Clin N Am 2013;22(4):569–80.
6. Sideli L, Murray R, Schimmenti A, et al. Childhood adversity and psychosis: a systematic review of bio-psycho-social mediators and moderators. Psychol Med 2020;50(11):1761–82.
7. Berry K, Barrowclough C, Wearden A. A review of the role of adult attachment style in psychosis: Unexplored issues and questions for further research. Clin Psychol Rev 2007;27(4):458–75.
8. Ball JS, Links PS. Borderline personality disorder and childhood trauma: evidence for a causal relationship. Curr Psychiatry Rep 2009;11(1):63–8.
9. Shah R, Zanarini MC. Comorbidity of borderline personality disorder: current status and future directions. Psychiatr Clin North Am 2018;41(4):583–93.
10. Baryshnikov I, Aaltonen K, Suvisaari J, et al. Features of borderline personality disorder as a mediator of the relation between childhood traumatic experiences and psychosis-like experiences in patients with mood disorder. Eur Psychiatry 2018;49:9–15.
11. Fusar-Poli P, Tantardini M, De Simone S, et al. Deconstructing vulnerability for psychosis: meta-analysis of environmental risk factors for psychosis in subjects at ultra high-risk. Eur Psychiatry 2017;40:65–75.
12. Peh OH, Rapisarda A, Lee J. Childhood adversities in people at ultra-high risk (UHR) for psychosis: a systematic review and meta-analysis. Psychol Med 2019;49(7):1089–101.
13. Green K, Browne K, Chou S. The relationship between childhood maltreatment and violence to others in individuals with psychosis: a systematic review and meta-analysis. Trauma, Violence, & Abuse 2019;20(3):358–73.
14. Birchwood M, Dunn G, Meaden A, et al. The COMMAND trial of cognitive therapy to prevent harmful compliance with command hallucinations: predictors of outcome and mediators of change. Psychol Med 2018;48(12):1966–74.
15. Spidel A, Lecomte T, Kealy D, et al. Acceptance and commitment therapy for psychosis and trauma: improvement in psychiatric symptoms, emotion regulation, and treatment compliance following a brief group intervention. Psychol Psychother 2018;91(2):248–61.
16. Dvir Y, Ford JD, Hill M, et al. Childhood maltreatment, emotional dysregulation, and psychiatric comorbidities. Harv Rev Psychiatry 2014;22(3):149–61.

17. Spidel A, Daigneault I, Kealy D, et al. Acceptance and commitment therapy for psychosis and trauma: investigating links between trauma severity, attachment and outcome. Behav Cogn Psychother 2019;47(2):230–43.
18. Tong J, Simpson K, Alvarez-Jimenez M, et al. Distress, psychotic symptom exacerbation, and relief in reaction to talking about trauma in the context of beneficial trauma therapy: perspectives from young people with post-traumatic stress disorder and first episode psychosis. Behav Cogn Psychother 2017;45(6):561–76.

Clinical Considerations in Internet and Video Game Addiction Treatment

David N. Greenfield, PhD, MS, ABPP[a,b,c],*

KEYWORDS

- Social media • Smartphone addiction • Online pornography
- Internet addiction treatment • Internet addiction • Process addiction
- Behavioral addiction • Video game addiction

KEY POINTS

- This article reviews etiologic and neurobiological antecedents to Internet and video game addiction.
- Internet and video game addiction is defined from a behavioral/process addiction framework as defined by The American Society of Addiction Medicine.
- Patient readiness for change, motivation, and harm reduction factors in Internet and video game addiction treatment are addressed.
- Unique and dynamic aspects of Internet, video game, and screen use that relate to addictive behavior are presented.
- Psychotherapeutic, pharmacologic, and strategic treatments are presented, along with the Center for Internet and Technology Addiction treatment model.

INTRODUCTION

To address the clinical issues and treatment strategies applicable to Internet and video game addiction (IVGA), a working definition, along with the identification of the unique behavioral aspects of Internet and screen use disorders is required. Common addictive patterns found specifically with Internet screen use often present with similar symptomatology to other behavioral and substance-based addictions, although severity and impairment vary widely.[1] There are numerous specific characteristics which appear

Child Adolesc Psychiatric Clin N Am 27 (2018) 327-344
https://doi.org/10.10167j.chc.2017.11.007 childpsych.theclinics.com
1056-4993/18/© 2017 Elsevier Inc. All rights reserved.
[a] The Center for Internet and Technology Addiction, 8 Lowell Road, West Hartford, CT 06119, USA; [b] Greenfield Pathway for Video Game and Technology Addiction, Lifeskills South Florida; [c] University of Connecticut, School of Medicine, Department of Psychiatry (former), Farmington, CT 06030, USA
* Corresponding author. The Center for Internet and Technology Addiction, 8 Lowell Road, West Hartford, CT 06119.
E-mail address: drdave@virtual-addiction.com

Child Adolesc Psychiatric Clin N Am 31 (2022) 99–119
https://doi.org/10.1016/j.chc.2021.09.003
1056-4993/22/© 2021 Elsevier Inc. All rights reserved.
childpsych.theclinics.com

to uniquely contribute to the addictive properties of Internet behavior. This article examines the etiologic and neurobiological antecedents to Internet and video game addiction, reviews the treatment literature, and presents the CITA model of treatment.

ADDICTION AND PROCESS/BEHAVIORAL ADDICTION DEFINED

Perhaps, the most comprehensive and descriptive definition of addiction is the one published by The American Society of Addiction Medicine (ASAM),[1] which captures both the neurobiological and behavioral components of addiction and along with disruption in the mesolimbic reward circuitry of the brain, creates behavioral and negative functional impacts in daily living (see definition of addiction in italics).

Abbreviations	
ADHD	Attention-deficit hyperactivity disorder
CBT	Cognitive behavioral therapy
IVGA	Internet and video game addiction
OCD	Obsessive-compulsive disorder
SSRI	Selective serotonin reuptake inhibitor
CITA	Center for Internet and Technology Addiction

Addiction is a primary, chronic disease of brain reward, motivation, memory, and related circuitry. Dysfunction in these circuits leads to characteristic biological, psychological, social, and spiritual manifestations. This is reflected in an individual pathologically pursuing reward and/or relief by substance use and other behaviors.

Addiction is characterized by inability to consistently abstain, impairment in behavioral control, craving, diminished recognition of significant problems with one's behaviors and interpersonal relationships, and a dysfunctional emotional response. As other chronic diseases, addiction often involves cycles of relapse and remission. Without treatment or engagement in recovery activities, addiction is progressive and can result in disability or premature death.[1]

Although premature death is a relatively infrequent consequence of IVGA, there are numerous psychological, behavioral, and physiologic sequelae to protracted Internet, video game, and screen use. In addition, excessive time spent online, regardless of Internet portal or content used, can create significant life impacts and imbalances.

Numerous anecdotal, clinical, and research studies describe various medical and physiologic sequelae, including elevated cortisol, hypertension, deep vein thrombosis, electrolyte imbalances leading to cardiac dysrhythmias, sleep disorders,[2] and obesity and related metabolic disorders.[3,4] Many of these health-related problems may be the result of extended sedentary behavior and poor diet. Most addictions, and IVGA is no exception, ultimately affect psychological functioning and life balance, notably the major spheres of living, including occupation and academics, social and interpersonal behavior, health and self-care, and motivation. With IVGA there are often presentations of comorbid and co-occurring psychiatric issues such as depression, social and generalized anxiety, attention-deficit hyperactivity disorder (ADHD), and affective dysregulation.[5]

Brain circuits implicated in the complex biobehavioral phenomenon of addiction include the ventral tegmental area/substantia nigra, amygdala, anterior cingulate, prefrontal cortex, and nucleus accumbens. These same circuits are also implicated in IVGA.[6,7] There seems little doubt as to the neurobiological similarities between substance-based and behavioral (or process) addictions.[6]

The ASAM addiction definition substantively captures the complex biopsychosocial interplay that defines addiction as a complex brain-behavior disorder. Research and historical analysis of addiction by Hari[8] and Alexander[9] strongly suggest social factors as a strong contributory factor for the development of an addiction to dopamine, innervating behaviors such as substance use and various behavioral addictions. We are hard-wired for social connection, and when access to such social connection is hampered by trauma, economic circumstances, and other psychological factors, engaging in intoxicating (dopamine innervating) substances or behaviors that modulates this need is enhanced. The maxim that social connection can serve to provide an antidote to addiction[8] seems relevant when examining the addictive process of Internet, video game, and social media—all of which provide pseudoconnection, while often simultaneously socially isolating the user. The irony that the Internet was initially hailed as a neuroprotective behavior to mitigate social isolation has proved problematic, especially when examining some of the most addictive forms of online content, such as social media, pornography, and video gaming.

A DIGITAL DRUG ADMINISTERED BY VIRTUAL HYPODERMIC

Some disagreement exists regarding the appropriate nosology for IVGA; however, there is considerable clinical and research data documenting the use, abuse, and addiction to the Internet and video gaming.[10–19] All forms of Internet content and video games are accessed easily via handheld devices, gaming consoles, and computers, as well as on smartphones and tablets, allowing significant ease of access,[20] thus increasing their addictive potential. Ease of access (or threshold reduction) is a significant variable relating to the addictive potential of a substance or a behavior, including Internet and video gaming, due to shorter latency between substance administration (or engaging in online behavior) and subsequent dopamine reinforcement—thus increasing addictive potential[20,21]; this is likely due to associated operant and classically conditioned features of tolerance and extinction resistance characteristic of addictions, including Internet-mediated addictions.[20]

The marked phenomenological overlap between Internet addiction, substance addiction, and pathologic gambling strongly suggests that a common neurobiological process involving affected reward circuits underlie these disorders and that the mesolimbic dopamine pathways likely represent a common pathway for neurobiological reinforcement and the biobehavioral addiction process from behavioral or pharmacologic stimuli. It seems that dopamine is the key neurotransmitter mediating pleasure, pain minimization, and reward deficiency in all additive processes.[5,22]

The use and abuse of content on the Internet (which increasingly involves the use of the smartphone Internet access portal) seems to hamper the ability to effectively manage time and attention, thus leading to hampered life-balance and other behavioral impacts. IVGA seems to affect motivation, reward, compulsion, memory, and often presents with co-occurring conditions, such as depression, social and generalized anxiety, and ADHD.

There are numerous factors that seem to contribute to the additive potential of the Internet. Several studies have found key factors that are associated with the compulsive use of the Internet and video games, including disinhibition, ease of access, content stimulation, synergistic amplification, boredom intolerance, dissociation (time distortion), perceived anonymity, and the variable activation of neurobiological reward pathways.[10,11,18,20,23]

Disinhibition

Disinhibition seems to allow users to express and experience themselves in a manner that is less affected by ego constraints, allowing them to take on alternate persona, roles, or behaviors. In our original research [11] we found that some of the variance accounting for this phenomenon was due, in part, to *perceived anonymity*. When on-line, it seems that it is easier to experience aspects of one's personality that might otherwise be less available in real-time communication; this may be due to inhibition of executive functions in the orbitofrontal area of the brain (which supports inhibitory processing). With all addictions the brain is essentially hijacked through the piggy-backing of primitive (survival-based) dopaminergic reward circuits, initially meant for insuring sustenance and procreation and that are supported by suppression of inhib-itory processes found in the frontal cortex; this makes sense from an evolutionary bio-logical perspective, as it enhances execution of quick-response, survival-based behavior. In essence, addiction may be seen as misplaced survival drives.

Ease of Access

Ease of access is a well-established contributory factor in all addictions; the ability to readily access intoxicating substances or behaviors increases the likelihood of compulsive or addictive use. Internet and video game availability functions as a neuro-biological trigger, facilitating activation of limbic brain pathways in a kindling-like manner; once ignited, the neuropathways and behavior patterns are activated and run on auto pilot. In addition, anticipatory dopamine innervation can occur simply by the visual cue of a computer, smartphone, or other Internet/video game device, thus priming brain reward circuits.

Content Stimulation

The Internet through its various access portals essentially becomes a virtual delivery mechanism for powerful and stimulating content. Video games, pornography, infotain-ment, social media, shopping, surfing/scrolling, You Tube, and gambling all have rein-forcing properties unto themselves. The power of the Internet is in part due to its unique, interactive ability to *rapidly deliver* content to the nervous system with *ease of access*, thereby creating a *reduced threshold* in accessing and experiencing such stimulating content.

Synergistic Amplification

The combination of stimulating content, delivered with rapid speed, produces a *syn-ergistic amplification* between *content* and the *Internet delivery mechanism*. Here, the whole is greater than the sum of its parts, and the combining of potent content with an accessible and efficient Internet delivery system produces an amplified and effective mood-altering dose.

Boredom intolerance

One of the most notable and frequent triggers of excessive Internet use, particularly on the smartphone, can be *boredom intolerance*. The ability to have a readily available Internet access portal, which is always on and accessible, facilitates the intolerance of being able to "do nothing"—for even brief periods of time. The more one surrenders to *screen simulation* and *attentional distraction*, the greater the neurobiological asso-ciation between their Internet/smartphone use and avoidance of unpleasant emotions or circumstances.

Dissociation (Time Distortion)

The experience of an altered perception of time is a ubiquitous experience of the Internet medium.[11,20,23] The Internet medium itself, combined with potentially stimu-lating content, alters the perception of time, thereby reflecting a psychoactive and mood-altered experience. There is a likely connection between the *distortion of time* and the experience of dopamine-mediated pleasure responses, which likely has its roots in the development of mammalian dopamine reward circuits.

Perceived Anonymity

This phenomenon is a significant marker for the online experience. Texting, instant messaging, direct messaging, surfing/scrolling, chat, email, social media posts, shopping, stock trading, online gambling, and pornography are frequently experienced as anonymous or quasi-anonymous, thus supporting the perception of a private communication and e-commerce experience. Nothing could be farther from the truth; in our early research[11,23] we found that the perception of *anonymity* was a significant factor in the attraction to and frequent use of the Internet. Users communicate, interact, and conduct business *as if* they are alone or in a way that reflects having a *personal* or *private* relationship with their device (and hence those whom they are communicating with through the Internet). Ironically, the Internet is perhaps the least anonymous of all communication mediums.

Activation of Neurobiological Reward Pathways

The Internet seems to activate the same mesolimbic reward pathways that are activated by various psychoactive substances and other addictive behaviors.[24] The efficient presentation of salient and rewarding stimuli in a variable format provides increase in extinction resistance and addictive potential of online behavior; anticipatory dopamine innervation (*The Maybe Factor*) further contributes to the powerfully captivating effects of the Internet medium with its correlated stimulating content. The short latency between the *click* or *tap* of a device and the rapid deployment of varied content provides a synergistically amplified experience. The faster an Internet device operates in accessing online content, the potentially greater the additive potential.

A VIRTUAL SLOT MACHINE

The Internet essentially functions as the *world's largest slot machine*. As noted, the Internet operates on a *variable ratio reinforcement schedule* due to the unpredictability in *what*, *when*, and *how desirable* the accessed content is. A slot machine operates similarly, where unpredictability (*The Maybe Factor*) keeps our brains tuned-in and vigilant; and encountering pleasurable (personally salient) stimuli facilitates a small and intermittent release of dopamine in the brain's reward center. Because these rewards are variable and unpredictable, frequent and compulsive checking of online and smartphone apps and content becomes a common occurrence. The behavior pattern of searching, scrolling, surfing, or scanning social media, such as You Tube, video games, pornography, shopping, news, information, and other forms of Internet content, becomes habitual and highly resistant to extinction. Checking phones can easily reach compulsive levels with hours of daily, dissociated use, regardless of the specific content accessed. Numerous studies[7,25] support that addictive Internet and video game use is associated with dopamine release in the mesolimbic system, which may lead to a desensitizing reduction in dopamine receptor expression (downregulation), reward deficiency syndrome, and hypofrontality.[5,20,25] There are numerous potential psychiatric sequelae for heavy Internet use, which may include reward deficiency–based depression, anxiety, impaired motivation, and inattention to balanced, real-time living behaviors.

The smartphone adds another dimension to Internet access with its frequent use of *notifications*. Users are constantly alerted via beeps, buzzes, and updates that inform them that *novel* information is waiting to be accessed; such notifications lead to the anticipation of *potentially desirable* content, thus providing a dopamine release. Anticipatory dopamine innervation is typically greater than subsequent reward, and it is the anticipatory reward that may contribute to the kindling or priming effect for further use of an Internet device, analogous with how one might keep playing on a slot machine after winning even a small amount. There is also evidence that suggests that the mere sight of a smartphone (along with notifications and rings) stimulates the release of the stress hormone cortisol, in turn triggering a self-medicating (stress-reducing) response by repeatedly checking their smartphone device.[3,4,26–28]

It seems that the most potent levels of dopamine innervation occur in conjunction with anticipation of reward, as compared with simply consuming the actual rewarding content itself—and anticipatory innervation may occur when one is *triggered* simply by the perceived availability of a screen device. The triggering effect from the presence of a smartphone may be analogous to the triggers, along with resulting urges and cravings, frequently seen with substance-based addiction behavior. The smartphone then may well be the *world's smallest slot machine*, fitting easily in one's purse or pocket and containing all the power and potency of a variably stimulating Internet access portal.

Smartphones can keep users on *automatic pilot*, responding to triggering stimuli on an automated, unconscious level, thus potentially inhibiting one from making healthy choices. Users may socially isolate, become intolerant of boredom, and maintain near-constant distraction levels with their devices—many addicted users become overstimulated, dopamine saturated, and attentionally impaired.

The new digital culture places less value on real-time experiences that are not broadcast or shared, as if our experiences have less value unless recorded, and then viewed, rated, and commented on by others. Echoic expressions of reflected self-esteem contribute to the phenomenon of social validation looping, where one repeatedly posts in order to receive social validation via likes, comments, and reposts; this process further contributes to the experience of fear of missing out, and the concern that one must continually update via social media while monitoring those updates, or one will fail to be noticed or socially included. Ironically, what we seem to be missing is the present-centered experience of our own lives and our own self-appraisal. Excessive Internet use may also contribute to health problems, including increased weight from sedentary behavior, eye strain, hand, finger, wrist, and upper back/neck strains, limited attentional capacity, hypertension, and stress from constant attentional vigilance.[29]

Compulsive smartphone use leading to elevated distractibility can also become a serious health threat; recent data[28,30] clearly demonstrate that excessive use often continues while users are driving their cars. Those who compulsively use smartphones while driving cause an alarming number of accidents, injuries, and deaths. Recent findings indicate that texting is not the only way smartphones distract drivers, because users engage in a variety of smartphone functions while driving.

TREATMENT CONSIDERATIONS

Treatment (as well as diagnostic nosology) of Internet addiction has not yet been standardized.[31–34] Historically addiction medicine has often lacked treatment standardization for many addictions,[35] and there remains some disagreement regarding the exact definition of Internet addiction, what to label it, and whether to classify it as a unified diagnosis or as distinct subdiagnosis[36]; regardless of these considerations, there is significant unmet public need for treatment services of screen-based behaviors.[33]

A significant demand for treatment of Internet addiction exists in the United States; prevalence statistics suggest a range of 0.5% to 12%.[33,34] Even greater demand exists in China, Taiwan, and South Korea, where the estimated prevalence among adolescents ranges from 1.6%[37] to 11.3%,[38] with some estimates placing 25% of youth as meeting criteria for IVGA. Despite considerable overlap in current measures for diagnosis, there is a lack of comprehensive and agreed-upon criteria; these factors contribute to the difficulty in precisely determining prevalence and therefore limit evaluating matched treatments. Treatment of addiction is often ultimately successful, but it frequently requires multiple treatment episodes before obtaining lasting sobriety; further, the very definition of *sobriety* with regard to IVGA is complicated in that abstinence is not fully attainable (as compared with substances) due to the necessary use of screen-based technologies for daily living.

SPECIFIED TREATMENT INTERVENTIONS

Once an adequate diagnosis of IVGA is made, the initial goal in treatment planning is to determine the level of motivation of the patient; the question of who is invested in the treatment process and outcome must be determined. In many cases, the patient may be a child, adolescent, or young adult, and treatment typically involves parents or loved ones; an attempt must be made to structure interventions based on the motivation and resources of the patient and family (or other support system).

It is also important to understand the developmental and psychosocial context of symptoms. Why is the patient presenting for treatment now? What developmental and biopsychosocial processes are ongoing for the patient? What stresses currently exist in patient's life? Are there social and relational problems that factor in?

Family reeducation is critical, especially around neurobiological education and helping parents understand that excessive or addictive use of the Internet or video games is not simply an act of willful defiance; such education is also helpful in reempowering the parents to help set appropriate boundaries, limits, consequences, and expectations. Parental involvement in treatment is essential for successful outcome when treating IVGA for younger patients. Strategies include boundaries and limit setting, as well as management of family technology through parenting skills—as well as with software and app-based blocking, limiting, and filtering. Modifying and controlling the patient's use or abuse pattern, marital factors (as there is often parental disagreement regarding screen use), medications, comorbidities, incentive induction, and positive reward transfer toward real-time living are key.

IMPLICATIONS OF CURRENT RESEARCH ON THE TREATMENT OF INTERNET AND VIDEO GAME ADDICTION AND RELATED INTERNET USE DISORDERS

IVGA often presents with *reward deficiency syndrome* caused by downregulation of dopamine receptors after excessive dopamine release secondary to exaggerated neurotransmitter interactions in the mesolimbic system.[39–42] Clinical considerations include screen-use history, tolerance, withdrawal, comorbidities, history of ADHD, possible genetic and epigenetic contributions, neurobiological mechanisms, and previous responses (if any) to treatment; it is suggested that behavioral (process) addictions such as IVGA resemble substance-based addictions and that excessive Internet use indeed presents with numerous features typically seen in the addiction spectrum. Winkler and colleagues[41] found that both pharmacologic and psychological treatments were effective in treating Internet addiction (time spent online, as well as symptoms of depression, and anxiety)—although there is still a dearth of data specific to appropriate patient-treatment matching.

COGNITIVE-BEHAVIORAL THERAPY

Numerous studies have suggested cognitive-behavioral therapy (CBT) is an effective treatment of Internet addictions.[32,43–49] Patients are trained to recognize cognitive and behavioral triggers that encourage self-medication using the Internet, screens, and video games and how to alter thoughts and behaviors to promote more moderated use.

A meta-review of Chinese Internet addiction studies[48] supported the relative efficacy of CBT, and most contemporary addiction treatment models have a strong CBT component. As Greenfield[50] notes, many, if not most, psychotherapeutic and behavioral interventions have cognitive-behavioral components, but addiction medicine heavily relies on psychoeducational strategies and in identifying the cognitive, emotional, and behavioral triggers and relapse antecedents.

Meta-analyses by King and Delfabbro[46] and others[47] found that cognitive-behavioral strategies are efficacious in managing IVGA; and similar results have been found in the treatment of substance abuse, especially for adolescents and young adults, for whom cognitive and psychoeducational approaches may be particularly effective.[51–53]

MOTIVATIONAL STRATEGIES: INTERVIEWING, ENHANCEMENT, AND HARM REDUCTION

Motivational interviewing and motivational enhancement are effective techniques to evaluate, establish, and enhance motivation for treatment and sobriety behaviors as well as in establishing the therapeutic alliance for treatment of addictions.[54] Patients seeking assistance for Internet-related disorders, as other addictions, have variable levels of readiness and motivation for change[55] and are frequently encouraged into treatment by a family member or loved one. This factor is particularly relevant in treating Internet and gaming addictions because these patients often lack an appreciation of the negative sequelae of their behavior and are therefore less motivated for clinical intervention. Successful treatment barriers can be exacerbated by a lack of a clinician's experience in treating IVGA and potential variability of professional acceptance of the disorder as a legitimate diagnosis. These factors, along with the view that the Internet and video games are *harmless entertainment*, can provide roadblocks in the treatment process.

MOTIVATIONAL INTERVIEWING AND MOTIVATIONAL ENHANCEMENT

People are generally better persuaded by the reasons which they have themselves discovered than by those which have come into the mind of others.
—*Blaise Pascal*

It is critical in the treatment of any substance or behavioral/process addiction that adequate treatment motivation exists. Many patients do not arrive for treatment at a high level of motivation, and therefore, attempts must be made to enhance treatment readiness and motivation and potentially enhance their willingness to receive help.[54]

It is important for the clinician to be aware of personal judgments, feelings, fears, and frustrations toward individuals experiencing Internet or video game addiction and to be conscious of a natural tendency to judge patient's addictive behaviors and actions. Being conscious of ascribing a negative prognosis in the face of a chronic, relapsing disorder such as an addiction is paramount to being clinically helpful. Some general guidelines are as follows:

- Become familiar with the neurobiology of addiction (and IVGA in particular) and help educate the patient (and family) to understand the process of IVGA. Many dealing with this issue do not know about the neurochemical and neurobiological factors associated with their illness.
- Learn to assess your patient's *readiness to change*, so you may apply appropriate motivational interviewing and motivational enhancement[56] interventions; it is important to remember that readiness to change and motivation are *not necessarily linear* and may wax and wane throughout the evaluation, treatment, and subsequent recovery process.
- Beware of cognitive dissonance, where we presume patient motivation (or lack thereof) and prognosis based on addiction-based behaviors.
- IVGA treatment and management can be challenging, but so are many chronic medical illnesses that we *still* attempt to treat.
- View addiction as any other chronic medical condition that may have exacerbations, remissions, and relapses—as well as recovery periods. Educate your patient about this recovery process and the psychological and biological factors found in addiction.
- Only 50% of the epidemiology for addiction seems to be genetic; the rest seems to be environmental/behavioral and epigenetic, which is the area where we, as clinicians, need to work.
- Remember (and remind the patient) that any improvement is a positive change and therefore reduces relative harm. Recovery from IVGA is *not all or none*, and small positive steps are always welcome.
- The longer the patient is able to moderate their use, the more likely that sustainable and balanced Internet and video game will occur.

READINESS FOR CHANGE AND TREATMENT

How many clinicians does it take to change a light bulb? One, but the light bulb must want to change.

The evaluation and management of patient motivation and readiness is a critical feature of Internet addiction treatment, just as it is with other addictions. Patients present at variable stages of readiness for change and recovery. The clinician must meet the patient with interventions appropriate to his or her level of motivation.[55] Stages of readiness for change are not always progressive, as patients frequently move back and forth among varying stages, requiring clinicians to maintain a flexible treatment approach. The stages of readiness and corresponding clinical goals are *precontemplation, contemplation, preparation, action, maintenance,* and *relapse.*

Precontemplation

In this early stage, the patient is not currently considering change. The clinician should validate a lack of readiness and normalize this experience. Clarify with the patient that the decision is theirs (although this becomes complicated when a parent is bringing a child or adolescent in for treatment). Encourage reevaluation of current behaviors and their consequences—without judgment. Stay curious and encourage the patient to be curious about themselves and about learning about their addiction. Foster exploration for the patient, not actions. Explain and personalize the risks of excessive Internet use through psychoeducation, including the neurobiological underpinnings of addiction. Encourage questioning of whether the patient has a problem by highlighting that other people (eg, parents, spouse, employer, friends) are concerned that they do.

Contemplation

In this stage, the patient is ambivalent about change or is "sitting on the fence." The patient in contemplation is probably not considering changing within the very near future. The clinician's goal is to validate their current lack of readiness and clarify that the decision regarding whether to change is theirs, although there may be natural consequences from their addictive behavior. Encourage evaluation of the pros and cons of behavior change and help to identify and promote positive potential outcome expectations.

Preparation

Patients at this stage have some experience with change and may be in the early stages of beginning to change addictive behavior: they are "testing the waters" and may be planning to act in the near future. Adolescents and young adults who are brought in for treatment by a family member are less likely to present at this stage. The clinician should help identify and assist in problem solving by helping them to remove possible obstacles for change to occur. Help the patient identify social supports with family and friends. Encourage small but attainable initial steps in the recovery process. Affirm that patient can access or develop the necessary skills and behaviors to change their Internet and video game use patterns.

Action

Patients at this stage are practicing new behaviors. Clinicians should focus on restructuring cues and triggers, as well as strengthening external supports, including family relationships and support groups. Bolster self-efficacy for dealing with material and emotional obstacles. Help combat feelings of longing, urges, cravings, and triggers for excessive Internet, video gaming, and screen use, emphasizing the long-term benefits of recovery and change. Highlight the positives of a balanced relationship with technology.

Maintenance

The patient has successfully changed their behavior and demonstrates a continued commitment to sustaining new (and healthier) behaviors; this outcome can occur at any point after beginning treatment, but typically after 6 months or more. Plan for supportive follow-up. Reinforce self-regulation and limit setting including internal rewards for positive behavior change and discuss coping with potential relapse. All these stages are not absolute or cumulative, and patients may move back and forth in their individual recovery readiness and stages of readiness for change.

Relapse

Here the patient has resumed previous Internet and video game behaviors. Clinicians should evaluate possible triggers contributing to the relapse including urges, cravings, and thoughts about the relapse. Develop or reaffirm a clear relapse prevention plan to be prepared for possible future relapses and lapses. Reassess motivation and possible barriers to mindful and moderated use and be on the lookout for negative cognitions and self-incrimination. Help the patient plan stronger coping strategies, as addiction is a chronic, relapsing disorder that can be progressive in severity, as well as cumulative in its recovery. Relapse is a normal part of the addiction recovery process, and Internet-based screen addictions are no exception.

Perhaps the greatest gift we can give in medicine is the installation of hope. Sometimes it is difficult for us as clinicians to feel hopeful or to adequately convey it to our patients—especially when we see our patients relapsing and experiencing negative life consequences. Medical compliance and treatment adherence is about 50%, yet in the treatment of addictions, we somehow expect greater treatment compliance, and when we do not see obvious progress, we might interpret this as a lack of motivation in our patients, which can then interfere with effective treatment.

ABSTINENCE VERSUS MODERATED AND MINDFUL TECHNOLOGY USE

Because we need to use the Internet for so many aspects of living, it is difficult to achieve complete abstinence with IVGA. The best option is *moderated*, *mindful*, and *value-based* use and to remove or limit the most problematic (triggering) content areas through external limits and controls. Modified use via behavioral and neurobiological disruption and repatterning (identifying and changing the trigger or urge response pattern) can begin to alter the well-established reward circuits. The goal is to eventually have positive reward transfer develop for real-time behaviors. Eye movement desensitization reprocessing has been a helpful tool in reducing urges and triggers,[35,57] as well as in treating concomitant social anxiety and social skills deficits.

Internet use disorder presents with a variety of unique characteristics in which addictive behaviors have become almost socially normative within our digital screen culture, further exacerbating denial among addicted users.[50] It seems we have come to accept the fact that we are all *somewhat* addicted to our screens, including video games and our smartphones. Internet entertainment (infotainment) reflect potentially addictive behaviors that have become acceptable within contemporary youth culture—the smartphone has rapidly become the dominant Internet access portal[58] and is often viewed as a necessary social tool and has been elevated to a *must-have* status.

A CLINIC-BASED TREATMENT PROGRAM FOR INTERNET AND VIDEO GAME ADDICTION AND EXCESSIVE SCREEN USE

Greenfield[50] developed a 7-step treatment process for IVGA and related screen use disorders. The model was developed for adolescents and young adults over a 20-year period while providing outpatient and intensive outpatient treatment of IVGA. This practical approach addresses treatment in a manner analogous to standard treatment protocols for other addictions, albeit with some variations, specific to screen behavior. This outline should not be treated as a lockstep or fixed treatment protocol but rather as a set of procedural guidelines. IVGA treatment must be flexible to be applied to the individual needs for each patient. Exacerbations, relapses, and treatment adjustments must be made throughout the process, and no 2 patients are alike; these guidelines can help inform the clinician on how to conceptually and clinically manage and treat IVGA and related screen use disorders.

The Center for Internet and Technology Addiction[37] uses a combination of psycho-education and neurobiological education, motivational interviewing, motivational enhancement, harm reduction, psychotherapy, pharmacotherapy, treatment of co-morbid and concurrent psychiatric issues, and eye movement desensitization reprocessing,[57] using a modified addiction management protocol.[55,56]

Patient Engagement and Rapport Building

In this critical stage, a collaborative treatment relationship is developed for the management and treatment of IVGA. This first stage of treatment is perhaps the most critical component of a successful treatment process, because without a collaborative relationship, treatment motivation, adherence, and compliance will be greatly reduced. It is key to building the treatment relationship and for assessing readiness for change, enhancing motivation, and increasing the patient's self-efficacy for potential positive change. Often, the addiction issues are not heavily addressed during the early phase of engagement.

Pattern Disruption

This phase is intended to disrupt the behavioral and functional aspects of the addiction and result in compulsive use patterns. The goal is to interrupt habitual coping, self-medication, and trigger-response loops and begin to allow new, more adaptive Internet and screen use to develop. Sometimes it is necessary to prescribe a period of relative abstinence (digital detox), with a particular focus on the most problematic content, for example, video gaming, pornography, social media, or shopping; very problematic content may need to be blocked and/or monitored at this stage in order to address the synergistic amplification of stimulating content and the Internet delivery mechanism. The goal is to help the patient begin to develop a more mindful, values-based use of the Internet and in so doing, begin the process of breaking neural pathways associated with their maladaptive use patterns. Because addiction involves disruptions of the mesolimbic reward circuitry, as well as antecedent and ritualistic behavioral patterns, we are attempting to shift this through actual pattern changes. We are using the neuroplastic and neurotrophic aspects of the brain-behavior interrelationship to gradually help rewire the addiction-behavior response pattern.

The goal is to begin to establish and strengthen new pathways and to begin to decrease the pattern of dopamine postsynaptic receptor (downregulation) associated with Internet-based addictive disorders. In so doing, we can begin to decrease the consequences of reward deficiency syndrome by minimizing excessive reward salience associated with screen use and slowly encouraging other forms of rewarding (dopaminergic) behavior. Ideally there will be the development of positive life consequences and rewards that are real-time oriented and naturalistic.

Trigger Identification

All addictions involve behavioral and situational triggers, which themselves have associated antecedents. It is critical to identify emotional and circumstantial triggers that kindle the additive cycle of behavior. Availability and opportunity (ease of access), boredom intolerance, anxiety (frequently social anxiety), and academic/work avoidance are common triggers, but there may be other triggers that are unique to the specific patient. The major treatment goal of this phase is for the clinician to help the patient *identify* the triggers for their compulsive screen use and to establish more moderated screen use habits. The goal is for the patient to develop increased self-awareness (and self-control) by identifying behaviors that exacerbate addictive patterns of use and by developing alternate real-time pleasure sources. Anticipation of triggers can become a method to counter-act anticipatory dopamine innervation from smartphone notifications (as well as other triggers), which can become a pathway to excessive screen use.

Management of Urges, Cravings, and Compulsions (Pharmacologic and Other Therapeutic Interventions)

In this treatment stage, psychoeducational and cognitive-behavioral strategies are most useful. The management of cravings to engage in excessive or pathologic Internet use involves an increased awareness of one's inner mood state as well as external environmental triggers.

Individuals experiencing Internet addiction are typically hyperfocused on screen access and content but unaware of their internal process. This lack of mindfulness, combined with time distortion/dissociation, perceived anonymity, and social media reliance, can impair real-time social connection—which may further exacerbate a desire to self-medicate. Nutritive social connection can be a partial antidote to IVGA, as the absence of real-time social connection can contribute to screen-induced social isolation. Internet addicts have little awareness of how much time they are spending online, thus further inhibiting self-reflection, trigger identification, and the monitoring of internal physiologic symptoms.

PHARMACOLOGY AND MEDICALLY AUGMENTED THERAPIES

Several recent studies have addressed the use of pharmacotherapy in the treatment of IVGA.[59–66] Antidepressants[59,61,63] and antipsychotics[59] have both been used with varying degrees of success, along with other pharmacologic agents. Evidence-based addiction medicine research has repeatedly demonstrated the need for the use of a combination of psychotherapeutic and psychoeducational approaches as the primary treatment of addiction, even while using medications. Pharmacotherapies may have promising usefulness as an adjunctive treatment of IVGA, as well as for management of comorbid symptomatology that is frequently found.

Several psychopharmacologic agents may be useful in medically augmented treatment of Internet addiction and related disorders, although research evidence regarding medication strategies is limited in both depth and breadth. Efficacy has been demonstrated to some degree for various antidepressants, opioid receptor antagonists and partial agonists, mood stabilizers, antipsychotics, glutamatergic drugs, W-methyl-D-aspartate receptor antagonists, and psychostimulants.[59–68]

The medication that has been studied most extensively for the treatment of IVGA is bupropion. A 6-week open-label trial of bupropion (sustained release) in 11 adult patients with IVGA was related to decreased craving for video games and cue-induced brain activity, Internet addiction scores, and time spend online.[65] It seems that the drug was effective, but the study noted limitations by its small sample size. A randomized, double-blind trial compared bupropion plus psychoeducation with placebo plus psychoeducation in 50 participants (13–45 year old) with excessive online gaming and major depressive disorder.[66] During the 8-week trial, those treated with bupropion showed improvement in depression and video game addiction symptoms and spent less time online than those treated with placebo. Bupropion seemed to be an effective adjunctive treatment of both depression and video game addiction in this study.

A third open-label clinical trial of 65 adolescents with comorbid major depressive disorder and video game addiction compared bupropion with combined bupropion plus group CBT.[45] After 8 weeks, both groups showed improvement, but the combination group showed greater benefit for video game addiction severity and life satisfaction compared with the medication-only group. This finding suggests that bupropion treatment of depression and video game addiction may be most effective when combined with CBT. There are obvious confounds in any study using antidepressant therapies for IVGA due to the frequent presentation mood inhibition due to reward deficiency syndrome.

One case report indicated that a patient with an Internet gaming addiction who was treated with escitalopram 30 mg for 3 months resulted in improved mood and a significant reduction in the drive to play online gaming, with a complete functional recovery.[61] An open-label trial of escitalopram (20 mg/d for 10 weeks) on 19 persons experiencing Internet addiction found significant decreases in weekly hours spent online and improvements in global functioning in 11 patients (64.7%).[61] At the end of the trial, subjects were blindly randomized either to continued escitalopram treatment or to placebo; both groups maintained gains made in the initial open-label treatment, but at the end of the double-blind phase there were no significant differences between the 2 groups. Larger controlled trials are clearly needed to investigate the efficacy of escitalopram and other selective serotonin reuptake inhibitors (SSRIs), as well as other psychopharmacologic agents for the treatment of IVGA.[63]

SSRIs may suppress inhibitory responses and the control of compulsive repetition, which likely explains their effectiveness in treating obsessive-compulsive disorders (OCDs). There also seem to be data indicating a higher lifetime prevalence of major depression in Internet addicts. Clinical studies have suggested a close relationship between affective dysregulation, impulsivity, and symptoms of the obsessive-compulsive spectrum, for which serotonergic drugs are known to be effective.[64,69,70] However, although effective in treating OCD, SSRIs have shown mixed results in some impulse control disorders, namely, pathologic gambling, kleptomania, and compulsive shopping (as well as Internet addiction).[62,67,68,70]

The augmentation of SSRIs with atypical antipsychotics for the management of refractory OCD is gaining increasing acceptance. IVGA has some features in common with OCD but seems to be a unique and distinct disorder with a specific symptom profile.

It has been hypothesized that quetiapine might be particularly useful for OCD[64] and may also be a safe and effective augmenting medication in cases with problematic Internet use. Atypical antipsychotics have been successfully used to remediate behavioral issues. In a review article Camardese and colleagues[62] proposed that SSRIs may potentially be efficacious in the treatment of IVGA and related disorders[62] associated with drug abuse, including impulsivity. Indeed, in our residential treatment program atypical antipsychotics have been found useful in management of anger and acting-out behaviors associated with withdrawal and dysregulation from excessive screen device use.

The role of psychostimulants in treatment of IVGA may be confounded by the frequent comorbidity of ADHD often seen in IVGAs. Indeed, it is uncommon for a patient to present with Internet addiction without preexisting or concomitant ADHD symptomatology; and pharmacologic interventions are often useful in addiction medicine as an adjunct for managing comorbid psychiatric symptoms, but less frequently for the pharmacologic management of urges, cravings, and triggers, which seems to be the case for psychostimulant management of IVGA. Many patients with IVGA who are treated with psychostimulants (without other targeted Internet addiction treatment) do not seem to benefit in terms of their addiction symptoms.

In an 8-week trial of methylphenidate treatment of children with ADHD who played online video games, Internet addiction score and Internet use times were significantly decreased. The changes in Internet addiction scores between the baseline and 8-week assessments were correlated positively with the changes in inattention scores and performance on the Visual Continuous Performance Test. This finding suggests that Internet video game play is directly related to ADHD severity and might be a means of self-medication or self-management for children with ADHD, which is reflected in the high rates of ADHD in patients with IVGA.[20,70] Perhaps the larger question is whether ADHD increases the incidence of IVGA or does IVGA increase levels of distractibility and decreased attention/concentration, further contributing to core ADHD symptoms, although there is likely to be an interactive and recursive process.

Opioid receptor antagonists inhibit dopamine release in the nucleus accumbens and ventral pallidum and other brain areas that mediate gratification, reinforcement, compulsion, and perseveration. Agents such as naltrexone have shown some clinical usefulness in the treatment of substance use disorders, gambling disorder, and klepto- mania and have also been considered for use in some behavioral addictions. However, research evidence regarding their effectiveness in IVGA are currently limited to case re- ports.[67] One case describes a successful treatment of online pornography addiction with naltrexone.[22,67] By blocking the capacity of endogenous opioids to trigger dopa- mine release in response to reward, naltrexone may, in theory, block the reinforcing na- ture of compulsive Internet and video game use,[69] Internet sexual activity, and theoretically other IVGA behaviors. Future research is needed to better assess the effectiveness of these and other pharmacologic agents in treating IVGA. For the time being medications seem to remain adjunctive to more effective and well-established psychotherapeutic and behavioral interventions, as described throughout this article.

Blocking, Monitoring, and Filtering

When dealing with substance-based addictions, addiction treatment often uses absti- nence from all abused substances (as well as other mood-altering substances). This goal seems appropriate, if not necessary, for effective substance use disorder treat- ment. With IVGA it is generally unrealistic (if not impossible) to avoid all Internet and screen use; many aspects of everyday life, including work, academics, banking, and most activities of daily living, are conducted online; Internet use is perhaps further exacerbated by our growing dependence on smartphones. The question remains whether it is possible to achieve abstinence from specific problematic areas of Internet use (such as video games, pornography, or social media) while continuing to use the Internet for necessary tasks in a mindful and moderate way.

An important goal for the treatment of Internet addiction is to monitor, limit, and possibly block specific *triggers*, including problematic content, apps, and Websites— as well as Internet content that serves as clear gateways to pathologic use. The initial goal is to detox (or at lease significantly limit) the most problematic content and then to reestablish screen technology use (possibly without the most triggering applications and Websites). It is sometimes possible to later reintroduce problematic content in a limited or modified manner with less risk of relapse; however, in the case of an addiction to video games, pornography, or social media it may be necessary to maintain ongoing abstinence. Many heavy Internet and video game users use games, apps, or content that can instigate addictive use and may thus need to be ultimately avoided. In addition, over- all daily screen use limits are almost always necessary in managing IVGA.

It should be noted that patients with a video game addiction often intersperse actual video gaming with watching recordings and streams of gaming on YouTube, Twitch, or other sites. This activity stimulates the addict and may trigger a craving to play, creating an increased likelihood for potential relapse. A qualified IT expert can help block, limit, or monitor such triggering sites or apps on the addict's devices, providing a buffer against triggering access to the most problematic sites and content, while allowing use of less problematic Internet use; this process can help create a delay that allows for the inhibitive orbitofrontal circuits to be more easily accessed, prevent- ing the near-instant gratification from stimulating and addictive online content. We have seen how addictive Internet content, once accessed, operates on a variable rein- forcement schedule, with ease-of-access often becoming an ignition point; IT blocks can serve to minimize potential relapse by disrupting extinction-resistant patterns.

An IT specialist can also set up monitoring software, providing the clinician with weekly reports detailing the patient's Internet use; in essence, this is an Internet abuse "toxicology screen," similar to a urine toxicology screen for substance-based addic- tions; such reports can also be used as a means of assessing the addict's overall use patterns and offer a preintervention (before treatment) analysis of content, apps, and websites that might need to be targeted, blocked or limited.

Care needs be taken not to assume that blocking, monitoring, or filtering a patient's online behavior will, on its own, be sufficient to treat Internet addiction. Often, patients' family members may attempt to manage their loved one's addiction via such blocks and filters, but IT strategies alone will likely fail unless part of a comprehensive treatment plan. The Internet addict is frequently more technologically sophisticated than their family and may also attempt to sabotage such technical efforts.

Studies imply that video game addicts undergo a similar mesolimbic reward activation from simply observing other people's play as when playing the games themselves.[22] As previously noted, many video game addicts, if blocked from playing their favorite games, will switch to other media modalities (eg, YouTube or Twitch) to watch others' gaming and experience gameplay vicariously or simply switch to binge-watching streamed television.

Reward deficiency syndrome

Addictions are, in part, supported and maintained by a reward deficiency syndrome, in which normal living seems flat and unrewarding compared with highly stimulating addictive behaviors. This desensitization (dopamine receptor upregulation) involves a weakening of circuits related to naturalistic reward, including social activities, work/academic reward, and delayed gratification of longer-term goals. Once an addict enters this state, previously reinforcing behaviors decrease and excessive amounts of time online increase. In addition, the addiction can be accompanied by a degree of developmental arrest with impairment of typical social, occupational, and academic milestones. Indeed, failure to launch is a frequent component of the IVGA patient, and patients typically need to resume healthy real-time living strategies to reintroduce naturalistic dopaminergic reinforcement.

In such cases of desensitization (upregulation of postsynaptic dopamine receptors) this can result in the weakening of circuits related to naturalistic rewards (eg, food, sex, self-care, socializing, work, or academic accomplishment). The Internet or video game addict may have a diminished capacity to enjoy such everyday pleasures and avoid delay of gratification, and the redevelopment of naturalistic reward stimulation therefore becomes essential in recovery. Nature abhors a vacuum, and as we decrease desensitized reward circuits, it is necessary to reestablish more naturalistic reward behaviors to serve as a prophylactic buffer in the recovery process.

Real-Time Living Strategies

A hallmark of successful treatment of any addiction is the instillation or reinstallation of normalized life skills and behaviors. The *Real-Time 100* involves a treatment strategy where the patient develops a list of 100 real-time behaviors (nonscreen based) that are introduced and used when urges, cravings, or triggers are noted; the idea is to slowly reintroduce normalized reward from real-time living and more naturalistic reward saliency back into the patient's life. Addiction creates an imbalance in functional and developmental tasks where the addictive behavior becomes the primary source of dopaminergic innervation in the nucleus accumbens and related brain reward structures. In the case of Internet and video game addicts, the inherit need for social competence, social validation, self-efficacy, accomplishment, and skills mastery becomes subsumed by Internet and screen-based activities.

RELAPSE PREVENTION

The goal of IVGA treatment is to maximize realistic sustainable recovery and maintain mindful moderation of technology use. For moderated use to continue, even after treatment has been completed, the clinician must help to inoculate the patient to relapse. The irony of relapse prevention is that one must acknowledge and assume potential relapse to help prevent it; and identifying triggers and situations, and rehearsing how these will be addressed when they occur, becomes a crucial part of any successful treatment.

INTERNET AND VIDEO GAME ADDICTION: A NEW DRUG OF CHOICE

Although a variety of therapeutic techniques have been presented for the treatment of IVGA, they are only at the beginning stages of identification, validation, and standardization. Although many of the general psychiatric and addiction treatments for Internet addiction are derived from established addiction medicine approaches, others are wholly novel and unique to these new digital drugs. Internet addiction treatment should rather be seen as a distinct subspecialty of addiction medicine requiring specialized behavioral/process addiction skills. Misdiagnosis is common, and many patients present for Internet addiction treatment only *after* numerous unsuccessful treatments failing to address the primary problem; frequently, treatment focuses solely on general psychiatric symptomatology, often with the erroneous bias that if such symptoms are corrected, compulsive screen use will diminish—this has not been supported at our clinic or in the literature. The treatment of Internet addiction has not yet attained the mature benchmark of evidence-based criteria, but research evidence continues to mount, and better designed and implemented research is on the horizon.

A common tenet in addiction medicine is that unless *addictive behavior* is addressed, treating comorbid psychiatric symptoms and disorders tends to be ineffective. Psychiatric conditions such as ADHD, depression, anxiety disorders, and autism spectrum symptoms may be premorbid or cooccurring and may also exacerbate as addiction sequelae.

An important perspective in treating Internet and video gaming addiction is that there is no need to reinvent the wheel. Many well-established addiction treatment protocols and techniques have proved effective in correcting similar disruptions of the reward pathways of the brain, with or without psychiatric comorbidities. Internet use disorders may be a new *drug of choice*, but numbing and self-medicating addictively are by no means new. We can draw from established substance use, alcohol use, and gambling disorder treatment protocols and therapies to help our patients who suffer from an addiction to the Internet and video games; we know what works in addiction medicine, and we know that addiction treatment often reflects an ongoing recovery process. With adequate patient motivation and targeted clinical care, healthier and sustainable technology use can be achieved and maintained over time.

ACKNOWLEDGMENTS

I acknowledge the patients at the Center for Internet and Technology Addiction, who over the last 25 years have guided the journey in treating this addiction. My 1999 study publication, *Psychological Characteristics of Compulsive Internet Use: A Preliminary Analysis*, represented early research to examine the addictive features of the Internet, and we have indeed come a long way since. I want to acknowledge all the researchers and clinicians who have advanced this field and who have continued to provide inspiration on the diagnosis and treatment of Internet and video game addiction. I would be remiss if I did not acknowledge those who were impactful in my early conceptualization of Internet addiction and its treatment. To the memory of my dear friend and colleague, Dr Alvin Cooper, for his early important work on the Internet affecting human sexuality and sexual behavior and who sparked my work in publishing on this subject—his *Triple A-Engine* concept was integral in my work. In memory of Dr Kimberly Young, whose pioneering work lit the pilot light of my own research and my first book, *Virtual Addiction*. And to the prolific body of work of my University of Connecticut, School of Medicine colleague, Dr Nancy Petry, whose scientific study of video game addiction helped move this field forward—her passing was a great loss. Lastly, to the late Dr Maressa Hecht Orzack, and our early publications on Internet sexual behavior.

DISCLOSURE

The author has nothing to disclose.

REFERENCES

1. Ries RK, editor. The ASAM principles of addiction medicine. 5th edition. Philadelphia (PA): Wolters Kluwer; 2014.
2. Foerster M, Henneke A, Chetty-Mhlanga S, et al. Impact of adolescents' screen time and nocturnal mobile phone-related awakenings on sleep and general health symptoms: a prospective cohort study. Int J Environ Res Public Health 2019;16(3):518.
3. Bibbey A, Phillips C, Ginty AT, et al. Problematic internet use, excessive alcohol consumption, their comorbidity and cardiovascular and cortisol reactions to acute psychological stress in a student population. J Behav Addict 2015;4(2): 44–52.
4. Reed P, Vile R, Osborne LA, et al. Problematic internet usage and immune function. PLoS One 2015;10(8):e0134538.
5. Greenfield DN. Overcoming Internet addiction for dummies. Hoboken (NJ): John Wiley & Sons; 2021.
6. Kuss DJ, Griffiths MD. Internet and gaming addiction: a systematic literature review of neuroimaging studies. Brain Sci 2012;2(3):347–74.
7. Kim SH, Baik S-H, Park CS, et al. Reduced striatal dopamine D2 receptors in people with Internet addiction. Neuroreport 2011;22(8):407–11.
8. Hari J. Chasing the scream. New York: Bloomsbury; 2015.
9. Alexander BK. Addiction: the urgent need for a paradigm shift. Subst Use Misuse 2012;47:1475–82.
10. Greenfield DN. The nature of internet addiction: psychological factors in compulsive Internet use. Paper presentation at the proceedings of the 1999 American Psychological Associa tion annual meeting, Boston (MA), August 20, 1999.
11. Greenfield DN. Psychological characteristics of compulsive internet use: a preliminary analysis. Cyberpsychol Behav 1999;2(5):403–12.
12. Greenfield DN. The nature of internet addiction: psychological factors in compulsive internet behavior. Journal of e.Commerce Psychol 2001;1.
13. Beard KW. Internet addiction: a review of current assessment techniques and potential assessment questions. Cyberpsychol Behav 2005;8:7–14.
14. Davis RA. A cognitive-behavioral model of pathological internet use. Comput Hum Behav 2001;17:187–95.
15. Griffiths MD. Does internet and computer "addiction" exist? Some case study evidence. Cyberpsychol Behav 2004;3(2):211–8.
16. King DL, Delfabbro PH. Understanding and assisting excessive players of video games: a community psychology perspective. Aust Community Psychol 2009;18: 62–74.
17. Young K. Caught in the net. New York: John Wiley; 1996.

18. Griffiths MD, Kuss DJ, Billieux J, et al. The evolution of internet addiction: a global perspective. Addict Behav 2016;53:193–5.
19. Griffiths M. Does internet and computer "addiction" exist? Some case study evidence. Cyberpsychol Behav 2000;3(2):181–8.
20. Greenfield DN. What makes internet use addictive?. In: Young K, Abreu CN, editors. Internet addiction: a handbook for evaluation and treatment. New York: Wiley; 2010. p. 135–53.
21. Allain F, Minogianis EA, Roberts DCS, et al. How fast and how often: the pharmacokinetics of drug use are device in addiction. Neurosci Biobehav Rev 2015;56: 166–79.
22. Jovic J, Dindic N. Influence of dopaminergic system on Internet addiction. Acta Med Medianae 2011;50(1):66.
23. Greenfield DN. Virtual addiction: help for netheads, cyberfreaks, and those who love them. Oakland (CA): New Harbinger Publications; 1999.
24. Duven E, Müller KW, Wolfling K. Internet and computer game addiction—a review of current neuroscientific research. Eur Psychiatry 2011;26:416.
25. Matthias E, Young KS, Elaier C. Prefrontal control and internet addiction: a theoretical model and review of neuropsychological and neuroimaging findings. Front Hum Neurosci 2014;8:375.
26. Kaess M, Parzer P, Mehl L, et al. Stress vulnerability in male youth with internet gaming disorder. Psychoneuroendocrinology 2017;77:244–51.
27. Lemieux A, Mustafa A. Stress psychobiology in the context of addiction medicine: from drugs of abuse to behavioral addictions. Prog Brain Res 2016;223:43–62.
28. Greenfield D. AT&T—it can wait survey of distracted driving. 2014. Available at: http://www.prnewswire.com/news-releases/are-you-compulsive-about-texting-driving-survey-saysyou-could-be-281586711.html; http://about.att.com/newsroom/compulsion_research_drivemode_ios_availability.html. Accessed October 17, 2017.
29. Stiglic N, Viner RM. Effects of screentime on the health and well-being of children and adolescents: a systematic review of reviews. BMJ Open 2019;9(1):e023191.
30. Greenfield DN. Driven to distraction: why we can't stop using our Smartphone's when driving. Keynote address at the 2017 Michigan traffic safety summit, Michigan State University, East Lansing (MI), March 23, 2017.
31. Przepiorka AM, Blachnio A, Miziak B, et al. Clinical approaches to treatment of Internet addiction. Pharmacol Rep 2014;66(2):187–91.
32. King DL, Delfabbro PH, Griffiths MD, et al. Assessing clinical trials of Internet addiction treatment: a systematic review and CONSORT evaluation. Clin Psychol Rev 2011;31(7):1110–6.
33. Byun S, Ruffini C, Mills JE, et al. Internet addiction: metasynthesis of 1996-2006 quantitative research. Cyberpsychol Behav 2009;12:203–7.
34. Griffiths MD. Internet and video-game addiction. In: Essau C, editor. Adolescent addiction: epidemiology, assessment and treatment. San Diego (CA): Elsevier; 2008. p. 231–67.
35. Greenfield DN. Internet use disorder: clinical and treatment implications of compulsive Internet and video game use in adolescents. Paper presentation at the Child & Adolescent Psychiatric Society of Greater Washington Spring symposium—Addictions and the Adolescent Brain, Suburban Hospital, Bethesda (MD), March 7, 2015.
36. Cash H, Rae CD, Steel AH, et al. Internet addiction: a brief summary of research and practice. Curr Psychiatry Rev 2012;8(4):292–8.

37. Kim K, Ryu E, Chon M, et al. Internet addiction in Korean adolescents and its relation to depression and suicidal ideation: a questionnaire survey. Int J Nurs Stud 2006;43:185–92.
38. Geng Y, Su L, Cao F. A research on emotion and personality characteristics in junior 1 high school students with Internet addiction disorders. Chin Ment Health J 2009;23:457–70.
39. Blum K, Chen AL, Braverman ER, et al. Attention-deficit-hyperactivity disorder and reward deficiency syndrome. Neuropsychiatr Dis Treat 2008;4(5):893–918.
40. Grant JE, Potenza MN, Weinstein A, et al. Introduction to behavioral addictions. Am J Drug Alcohol Abuse 2010;36:233–41.
41. Winkler A, Dorsing B, Rief W, et al. Treatment of Internet addiction: a meta-analysis. Clin Psychol Rev 2013;33:317–29.
42. Du Y, Jiang W, Vance A. Longer term effect of randomized, controlled group cognitive behavioral therapy for Internet addiction in adolescent students in Shanghai. Aust N Z J Psychiatry 2010;44:129–34.
43. Jorgenson AG, Hsiao RCJ, Yen CF. Internet addiction and other behavioral addictions. Child Adolesc Psychiatr Clin N Am 2016;25(3):509–20.
44. Jager S, Müller KW, Ruckes C, et al. Effects of a manualized short-term treatment of internet and computer game addiction (STICA): study protocol for a randomized controlled trial. Trials 2012;13(1):1.
45. Kim SM, Han DH, Lee YS, et al. Combined cognitive behavioral therapy and bupropion for the treatment of problematic on-line game play in adolescents with major depressive disorder. Comput Hum Behav 2012;28(5):1954–9.
46. King DL, Delfabbro PH. The cognitive psychology of internet gaming disorder. Clin Psychol Rev 2014;34:298–308.
47. Young KS. CBT-IA: the first treatment model for internet addiction. J Cogn Psychother 2011;25:304.
48. Liu C, Liao M, Smith DC. An empirical review of internet addiction outcome studies in China. Res Soc Work Pract 2012;22(3):282–92.
49. King DL, Delfabbro PH, Griffiths MD, et al. Cognitive-behavioral approaches to outpatient treatment of internet addiction in children and adolescents. J Clin Psychol 2012;68(11):1185–95.
50. Greenfield DN. Internet and technology addiction: are we controlling our devices or are they controlling us? Keynote address at the proceedings of the National Association of Social Workers—South Dakota annual meeting, Sioux Fall (SD), March 17, 2016.
51. Young K. Cognitive behavior therapy with Internet addicts: treatment outcomes and implications. Cyberpsychol Behav 2007;10:671–9.
52. La Salvia TA. Enhancing addiction treatment through psychoeducational groups. J Subst Abuse Treat 1993;10:439–44.
53. Botvin GJ, Baker E, Filazzola AD, et al. Cognitive-behavioral approach to substance abuse prevention; a one-year follow up. Addict Behav 1990;15:4743.
54. Miller WR, Rollnick S. Motivational interviewing: helping people change. New York: The Guilford Press; 2013.
55. Prochaska JO, DiClemente CC, Norcross JC. In search of how people change: applications to the addictive behaviors. Am Psychol 1992;47:1102–14.
56. Marlatt GA. Taxonomy of high-risk situations for alcohol relapse: evolution and development of a cognitive-behavioral model. Addiction 1996;91(Suppl):37–49.
57. Shapiro F. Eye movement desensitization and reprocessing: basic principles, protocols, and procedures. 2nd edition. New York: The Guilford Press; 2001.

58. Pew Research Center, June 2019, Mobile Technology and Home Broadband, 2019.
59. Atmaca M. A case of problematic internet use successfully treated with an SSRI-antipsychotic combination. Prog Neuropsychopharmacol Biol Psychiatry 2007; 31(4):961–2.
60. Moreira FA, Dalley JW. Dopamine receptor partial agonists and addiction. Eur J Pharmacol 2015;752:112–5.
61. Camardese G, De Risio L, Di Nicola M, et al. A role for pharmacotherapy in the treatment of internet addiction. Clin Neuropharmacol 2012;35(6):283–9.
62. Camardese G, Leone B, Walstra C, et al. Pharmacological treatment of Internet addiction. In: Montag C, Reuter M, editors. Internet addiction. Studies in neuro–science, psychology and behavioral economics. Springer International Publishing; 2015. p. 151–65.
63. Dell'Osso B, Hadley S, Allen A, et al. Escitalopram in the treatment of impulsive-compulsive Internet usage disorder: an open-label trial followed by a doubleblind discontinuation phase. J Clin Psychiatry 2008;69(3):452–6.
64. Goddard AW, Shekhar A, Whiteman AF, et al. Serotoninergic mechanisms in the treatment of obsessive-compulsive disorder. Drug Discov Today 2008;13(7–8): 325–32.
65. Han DH, Hwang JW, Renshaw PF. Bupropion sustained release treatment decreases craving for video games and cue-induced brain activity in patients with Internet video game addiction. Exp Clin Psychopharmacol 2010;18(4): 297–304.
66. Han DH, Renshaw PF. Bupropion in the treatment of problematic online game play in patients with major depressive disorder. J Psychopharmacol 2012; 26(5):689–96.
67. Bostwick JM, Bucci JA. Internet sex addiction treated with naltrexone. Mayo Clin Proc 2008;83(2):226–30.
68. Grant JE, Kim SW, Hollander E, et al. Predicting response to opiate antagonists and placebo in the treatment of pathological gambling. Psychopharmacology (Berl) 2008;200(4):521–7.
69. Besson M, Belin D, McNamara R, et al. Dissociable control of impulsivity in rats by dopamine D2/3 receptors in the core and shell subregions of the nucleus accumbens. Neuropsychopharmacology 2010;35:565–9.
70. Bernardi S, Pallanti S. Internet addiction: a descriptive clinical study focusing on comorbidities and dissociative symptoms. Compr Psychiatry 2009;50(6):510–6.

Desensitization and Violent Video Games

Mechanisms and Evidence

Jeanne Funk Brockmyer, PhD

KEYWORDS

- Video games • Violence • Desensitization • Media violence • Aggression • Empathy
- Moral reasoning • fMRI

KEY POINTS

- Desensitization, the reduction of cognitive, emotional, and/or behavioral responses to a stimulus, is an automatic and unconscious phenomenon often experienced in everyday life.
- It has been proposed that exposure to violent media, especially violent video games, may cause desensitization to real-life violence.
- Desensitization of violence blocks empathy. If empathy is blocked, moral reasoning will not occur, impeding prosocial and allowing negative responding.
- Representative data were reviewed to examine links between exposure to violent video games and desensitization to violence in children and adolescents.
- It was concluded that exposure to violent video games increases the risk of desensitization to violence, which in turn may increase aggression and decrease prosocial behavior.

THE PHENOMENON OF DESENSITIZATION

Desensitization, the reduction of cognitive, emotional, and/or behavioral responses to a stimulus, can be a powerful therapeutic tool when it is intentional. Desensitization is also an automatic, unconscious phenomenon often experienced in typical, everyday life experiences. This can be best demonstrated through the following exercise: Think back about a traumatic event you learned about, perhaps the first mass shooting in your lifetime. For some, it may be the 1999 Columbine school shooting, for others, the 2007 Virginia Tech mass shooting. There are many. Try to recall your thoughts and emotional reactions. Now consider your response to one of the myriad subsequent mass shootings. Most likely this response is not as intense as your reaction to the original one. This change reflects unconscious, adaptive, and normal

The author has nothing to disclose.
Department of Psychology, University of Toledo, MS 948, 2800 West Bancroft, Toledo, OH 43606-3390, USA
E-mail address: jeanne.brockmyer@gmail.com

Child Adolesc Psychiatric Clin N Am 31 (2022) 121–132
https://doi.org/10.1016/j.chc.2021.06.005
1056-4993/22/© 2021 Elsevier Inc. All rights reserved.

desensitization. Repeated exposures to similar traumas normally result in a reaction that is less intense than the reaction to the initial trauma. In fact, those whose reactions do not habituate to repeated similar traumatic exposures may have increased susceptibility for developing some form of psychopathology.

However, unconscious desensitization can also be maladaptive. For example, researchers have found that children who are exposed to high levels of community violence come to view violence as an ordinary part of life and may act accordingly.[1,2] This world view represents a form of desensitization to violence. Similarly, exposure to media violence and especially video game violence has been identified as potentially desensitizing for children and adolescents.[3]

This article first examines the pathway by which desensitization to violence may theoretically lead to a failure of empathy, which obstructs moral reasoning, blocking prosocial responding and allowing negative responding. Then, representative research evidence is discussed, demonstrating that exposure to video game violence can be a risk factor for desensitization to violence. Finally, clinical implications and recommendations are presented.

EMPATHY

Because empathy has been studied by many different disciplines, it has been difficult to agree on a specific definition of empathy. It is generally accepted that empathy is best understood in terms of two components: emotional empathy and cognitive empathy.[4] Emotional empathy is the actual experience of the feelings of another while cognitive empathy is the ability to take the perspective of another person. Feeling empathy alerts an individual to the moral relevance of a situation and activates the process of moral reasoning.

Development of empathy

Humans are born with the capacity for empathy. Newborn nurseries are famous for sequential crying: One crying baby tends to trigger crying in the others. The development of true empathy requires a certain sequence of life experiences. First, it is critical for infants to have reliable, warm, responsive parenting. Later in childhood, the development of complexity in emotion, cognition, and motor skills leads to the capacity to develop basic prosocial behavior. As development proceeds, empathy and empathic responding are strengthened through modeling, direct teaching that identifies the perspective and feelings of others, and reinforcement of empathic choices. An accumulation of such experiences supports the development of mature empathy.[5]

MORAL REASONING

Moral reasoning is a psychological process that guides behavioral choice. Moral reasoning continually undergoes developmental transformations.[5] For example, preschoolers are most likely to reason simplistically, in ways that primarily benefit themselves. By elementary school age, moral reasoning begins to involve concern for peer and adult approval, but children still tend to judge situations in simplistic "good" and "bad" terms. In adolescence, mature moral reasoning, which includes abstract concerns about justice and caring for others, begins to emerge. When fully mature, moral reasoning includes behavioral self-monitoring. At this point, when personal moral standards are violated, this results in self-reproach and distress.

Mature empathy is necessary for the internalization and activation of moral reasoning.[6,7] As mature empathy develops, it becomes an important prompt for initiation of moral reasoning processes and thus an important motivator for prosocial behavior. Feeling empathy alerts an individual to the moral relevance of a situation and triggers moral reasoning processes that aid in choosing a behavioral response. Failure to empathize may block moral reasoning and prosocial responding.[8]

Moral disengagement

In a situation where an individual is experiencing distress or pain, typically an empathic response by another will trigger that person's moral reasoning, leading to a prosocial helping response. If empathy is not triggered, moral reasoning will not be activated, and moral disengagement may occur. Moral disengagement is a psychological process by which individuals separate moral standards from actions, rationalizing immoral behavior.[9] Consequently, moral disengagement permits immoral behavior without self-judgment or anxiety. Signs of moral disengagement include attributing one's immoral actions to external factors, misperceiving the importance and consequences of one's antisocial actions, and dehumanizing or disparaging the victim of the negative behavior. Moral disengagement is a sign of impaired moral reasoning and may reflect desensitization.[9]

Moral disengagement may explain why otherwise gentle and law-abiding individuals enjoy playing violent video games.[10] Violent video games typically have many prompts that promote automatic moral disengagement. These include justification of violence, dehumanization of game victims, and distorted portrayal of consequences, particularly the consequences of violence.[11] Moral rationalization, another aspect of moral disengagement, is the act of reasoning that engaging in extremely violent actions is all right because "it is just a game." With these psychological mechanisms readily available, virtual violence simply does not feel wrong to the player, and as violent actions are justified, violent video game play is guilt-free. Importantly, research suggests that when violence is not justified, players do feel guilty, most likely because unjustified violence triggers an empathic response for victims, this triggers the moral reasoning process, and moral disengagement does not occur.[9]

VIOLENT VIDEO GAMES AND DESENSITIZATION TO VIOLENCE

Media permeate the daily life of most American children and adolescents, and video games account for a large portion of media exposure. According to the Entertainment Software Association (ESA), the body that developed and maintains the video game rating system, total video game sales in 2018 exceeded $44.4 billion.[12] Many games that are popular with children and adolescents have violent content. The Entertainment Software Rating Board (ESRB) is the arm of the ESA that actually rates games.[13] Age recommendations, content descriptors, and a listing of "interactive" (game purchases, how users can interact) elements are provided. According to 2020 research by Norton, although most games are rated by the ESRB as being for everyone, 49% of video games have some type of violent content[14] (**Fig. 1**). A 2013 report by the Kaiser Family Foundation indicated that nine out of ten (89%) of the top-selling video games contained violence; in addition, about half of all games contained serious violence, and 17% featured violence as the primary focus of the game.[15]

After a careful literature review that included four meta-analyses, the American Psychological Association's Task Force Assessment of Violent Video Games concluded that "the use of violent video games results in increases in overall aggression as well as increases in the individual variables of aggressive behaviors, aggressive cognitions, aggressive affect, desensitization, physiologic arousal, and decreases in empathy (p. 142)."[16] This has been demonstrated in multiple single studies, including longitudinal work, and in several meta-analyses.[17–19] It should be mentioned that one group of

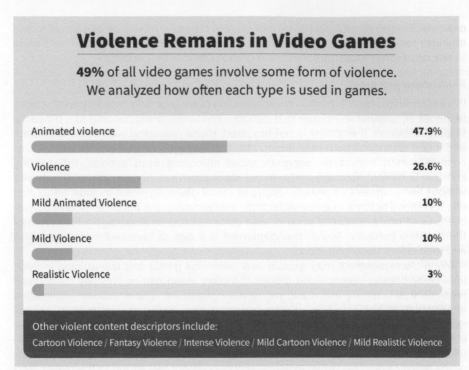

Violence Remains in Video Games

49% of all video games involve some form of violence.
We analyzed how often each type is used in games.

Animated violence	**47.9%**
Violence	**26.6%**
Mild Animated Violence	**10%**
Mild Violence	**10%**
Realistic Violence	**3%**

Other violent content descriptors include:
Cartoon Violence / Fantasy Violence / Intense Violence / Mild Cartoon Violence / Mild Realistic Violence

Fig. 1. Content analysis of rated video games. (NortonLifeLock (2021, Jan. 14). 2020 video game ratings in review, and what they mean to gamers. https://us.norton.com/internetsecurity-kids-safety-video-game-ratings.html.)

meta-analysis researchers came to a different conclusion, that there is no such relationship.[19] However, work by Mathur and VanderWeele[20] elegantly explained these apparently inconsistent results as actually being a function of the approach to statistical analysis of the data, concluding that results of the three meta-analyses they studied, including the one with null interpretation of findings,[19] were actually in agreement that violent video games have a small though consistent effect on aggressive behavior.

RESEARCH ON VIOLENT VIDEO GAMES AND DESENSITIZATION TO VIOLENCE

Measurement issues impeded early research on violent video game–related desensitization in part because, by definition, desensitization is the absence of an expected response.[21] Several short-term and a handful of longer term studies of video game–related desensitization are now available using multiple research modalities. In addition to survey and behavioral studies, current research takes advantage of the fact that cognitive and emotional desensitization may be seen in diminished physiologic arousal. The following is guided by this principle: In research on real-world phenomena, such as media effects, a convergence of evidence from a variety of research approaches is the gold standard for drawing conclusions about whether or not the evidence supports an effects model.[22] Representative research is presented in the following parts of the article.

Questionnaires

Questionnaires are typically used to collect large amounts of information from cross-sectional samples, often based on self-report. Some questionnaire studies have examined exposure to violent video games and characteristics such as empathy and attitudes toward violence.[21]

The development of positive or neutral attitudes toward violence is influenced by many factors, including exposure to violence in real life and in entertainment media. Proviolence attitudes may play an important role in the translation of negative cognitions and affect into behavior.[23] Empathy and attitudes toward violence are components of the process of moral reasoning that may reflect both emotional and cognitive desensitization, with empathy being decreased and proviolence attitudes being strengthened.[21]

Several survey-based studies have examined empathy and attitudes toward violence in relation to exposure to violent video games. For example, fourth and fifth graders (N = 150; 68 girls) completed measures of different forms of real-life and media violence exposure, empathy, and attitudes toward violence. Only exposure to video game violence was associated with (lower) empathy. Both video game and movie violence exposure were associated with stronger proviolence attitudes.[24] In a survey of 312 Chinese adolescents (35% female), Wei[25] found that a higher level of exposure to violent video games online was associated with lower empathy and stronger proviolence attitudes, with stronger effects for males than for females. The author concluded that these results are consistent with the desensitization theory. A large sample of seventh and eighth graders (N = 1237; 51.5% female) in Germany were surveyed by Krahe and Moller[26] twice over a 12-month period. Self-reports of habitual violent media usage at time 1 were related to self-reports of lower empathy and higher physical aggression at time 2, possibly reflecting desensitization to violence.

Behavioral research

Behavioral research examines behavioral changes that occur after exposure to violent video games, often using both questionnaires and direct behavioral measurement. For example, Grizzard and colleagues[27] examined desensitization by measuring guilt over five sessions of violent video game play. Players represented either a United Nations soldier or a terrorist on alternate days over 4 days of play. On the fifth day, everyone played a different violent game, taking the role of a terrorist. After each session of playing, participants completed measures of guilt about their violent choices during game play. The researchers found that repeated exposure to the first violent game decreased this game's ability to cause guilt over the 4-day period. More importantly, this decline in guilt about using violent actions in a game was generalized to the second game even though it was only played once, suggesting desensitization to the violence.[27]

In research combining questionnaire and behavioral methods, Bartholow and colleagues[28] examined, among other variables, the possible mediating role of empathy in the relationship between exposure to violent video games and aggressive behavior. Male college students (N = 92) completed questionnaires and played a violent or nonviolent video game. Regarding desensitization, those with high prior exposure to violent video games had higher levels of aggression than those with less exposure. Empathy was one mediator of this effect. German researchers found that subjective evaluation of in-game violence was affected by playing (as opposed to watching) a violent video game for 30 high school and college students (50% female).[29] They suggested that this could indicate an immediate desensitization effect.

Violent video games and real-world behaviors

Researchers have also examined associations between exposure to violent video games and documented negative real-world behaviors. For example, DeLisi and colleagues[30] examined associations between violent video game play and measures of delinquent behavior in a sample of institutionalized juveniles (N = 227; 45% female) aged 14 to 18 years. Using interview and survey methods, the researchers found that frequency of violent video game play and a measure of liking for violent games were significantly associated with general and violent delinquency after controlling for the effects of screen time, years playing video games, age, gender, race, delinquency history, and psychopathic personality traits. Although desensitization to violence was not measured directly, the juveniles all had histories of criminality, and many had histories of violent behavior.

Canadian researchers surveyed about 800 parents and their children (age 10–17 years; about half female).[31] Their online survey assessed bullying behavior (reported by both children and parents) and the child's three favorite games, which were coded by the researchers for level of violence. For male and female children, general bullying and cyberbullying were related to preferences for playing violent video games, based on the parents' and children's responses. This may reflect desensitization to the suffering of others.

Psychophysiologic measures

A variety of basic psychophysiologic measures have been used to examine short- and long-term effects of exposure to violent video games, including skin conductance,[32] heart and respiratory rate,[32,33] and pupillary response.[34] Most research with these measures demonstrates desensitization effects. There is emerging evidence from research using event-related potential (ERP) and functional magnetic resonance imaging (fMRI) that exposure to violent media may be linked to decreases in the activity of brain structures needed for the regulation of aggressive behavior and to increases in the activity of structures needed to carry out aggressive plans.[35]

Neurodevelopment is a continuous, dynamic process that is sequential and use-dependent. When an individual repeatedly engages in repetitive, structured, patterned activities, permanent changes in brain reactivity may occur.[36] In the case of exposure to violent video games, disuse-related extinction of the empathy precursor to moral reasoning could result. In that case, the distress response to violence would not be triggered, indicating desensitization. A body of research using ERP is sampled in the following paragraphs. Contemporary research appears to be focusing on fMRI research, and this is also discussed in the following paragraphs.

Event-related potential

ERP has been a widely used measure in research on violent video game players and desensitization for several years. Smaller P3 amplitudes to presentations of violent images after violent video game play are thought to reflect deficits in the aversive motivational system, in other words, desensitization. For example, in one study, 70 young adults (46% female) reported their history of violent video game play, then played either a violent or nonviolent video game, and then viewed violent and nonviolent photos while having brain activity measured.[37] Comparing participants with less prior exposure only, those who played a violent game had a lower P3 response than those who played a nonviolent game. This suggests that playing the violent game desensitized the low-exposure players to violence in the photos. Compared with low-exposure participants, high-exposure participants had a lower ERP response to violent images, which may indicate long-term desensitization.

Jabr and colleagues[38] used a rapid serial visual presentation (RSVP) task to examine N1 and P3 ERP activation differences between 67 (43 female) adult video game players and nonplayers while viewing a series of violently aversive and neutral pictures selected from the International Affective Pictures System (IAPS).[39] They also completed a measure of aggressive tendencies. The N1 ERP is associated with selective attention, and the RSVP task is an attentional blink paradigm. The attentional blink phenomenon occurs when the second of two targets cannot be detected when it is presented very closely to the first. In the present context, an attentional blink is generated when an emotionally challenging stimulus requiring substantial attentional resources is presented shortly before a stimulus requiring action. The second stimulus is "blinked" (not readily perceived) because most attentional resources have been used by the first target. In the present study, participants had to recall the neutral picture and push a button to indicate what was recalled. Results indicated that violent game players had blunted P3 amplitudes, compared with nongamers, indicating desensitization. Gamers had more negative N1 activation than nongamers, particularly for violent stimuli, suggesting a selective attention bias in favor of violent stimuli.[38]

Although most published ERP studies identify desensitization as related to violent video game exposure, one ERP study that did not support a desensitization effect was found. Goodson and colleagues[40] examined the P3 component of 87 adult volunteers (49 female) in response to violent stimuli. Participants completed a questionnaire about experience with violent video games. Their self-report to a dichotomous question indicated that 53 had experience (amount not given) playing violent video games, while 34 had no experience with such games. Participants first viewed both violent and neutral images from the IAPS while ERPs were recorded. They then played a violent video game. Then participants again viewed IAPS pictures while ERPs were recorded. Comparing those with a self-reported history of playing violent video games to those with no history, there was no difference in P3 activation to the stimuli. However, the authors not only questioned the validity of the P3 as a measure of desensitization to violence but also noted that the data actually appeared to come from one sample, not two unique groups as assumed by the research. This may have been methodological (eg, no measure of amount of prior experience with violent video games).

Functional magnetic resonance imaging
While most ERP research does identify some desensitization effect, results of fMRI research are mixed. Nine relevant publications were identified from a search of MEDLINE/PubMed and PsychInfo. Four identified a desensitization effect,[33,41–43] while five[44–48] did not. **Table 1** was created to understand possible methodological differences that could account for these inconsistencies. Most of the table headings are self-explanatory, but the comparison group column requires additional description. The term "By History" means that the sample was divided into groups based on the game-playing history and preference as provided by the participant. It is worth noting that four of the five studies not finding a desensitization effect assigned participants by history, which may not be accurate. The column labeled "Short or Long-Term" also deserves explanation. This column refers to whether the desensitization effect is based on a short-term, experiment-based exposure to a violent video game or to a long-term exposure, as reported by the participant usually over the participant's lifetime. The one exception to this explanation is research by Kuhna and colleagues[45] who used a longitudinal experimental design. These researchers asked participants to play either the same violent game, the same nonviolent game, or serve as a no-game participant 30 minutes daily (at home, unsupervised) for 8 weeks. fMRI scanning was performed before game-playing, at the end of the 8 weeks of play, and 16 weeks after the experiment began. A weakness of the study is that the researchers assume that participants complied with the directions, but there was no way to be certain of the dose of gaming

Table 1
Violent video games and desensitization: comparison of fMRI research with positive versus negative findings

Researchers, Year	Game Experience Assessed	Gender	N	Comparison Group	Adult, Child, or Adolescent	Short or Long Term	Primary Stimulus For fMRI	When Scanned
Relationship identified								
Weber et al,[43] 2006	Yes	Male	11	No	Adult	Short	Game	During game
Montag et al,[35] 2008	Yes	Male	40	Case control	Adult	Long	Pictures Realist/Non Pleasant/Non	No game During viewing
Guo et al,[42] 2013	No	75% Female	30	Random assign	Adult	Short	Pictures Painful/Non	No game During viewing
Gentile et al,[41] 2016	Yes	Male	13	By history	Adult	Short	Games Viol/Non	During game
Relationship not identified								
Regenbogen et al,[46] 2010	Yes	Male	22	By history	Adult	Short	Video clips Realistic/Non Violent/Non	No game During viewing
Szycik et al,[47] 2017	Yes	Male	30	By history	Adult	Long	Line drawings Neg/Neutral Emo Interact or Not	No game During viewing
Szycik et al,[48] 2017	Yes	Male	56	By history	Adult	Long	Photos Neg/Pos/Neutral	No game
Gao et al,[44] 2017	Yes	Male	35	By history	Adult	Long	Computer-photos Painful/Non	No game
Kühna et al,[45] 2018	No	53% Female	80	Random assign	Adult	Long, 16 wk Unsupervised	Photos Realistic/Non Pain/No pain	Before/after any play (8 wk) During viewing; 4 mo after beginning experiment

received by each participant. It seems likely that this could explain why no desensitization effect was identified. Scanning for the other four studies that did not identify a desensitization effect was carried out without any in-experiment game-playing. Additional fMRI research is needed that uses best experimental practices (eg, randomized controls, attention to prior game experience, verifiable doses of game play).

SUMMARY

As noted earlier, in research on real-world phenomena, a convergence of evidence from a variety of research approaches is needed before drawing conclusions about whether or not the evidence supports anticipated effects. In the area of the effects of exposure to violent video games, most evidence is converging toward desensitization although additional fMRI research is needed, particularly with children.

These findings do not mean that every player of violent video games will be desensitized. A risk and resilience approach suggests that exposure to violent video games will increase the relative risk of desensitization to violence, with those who already have increased vulnerability being at greatest risk.[49,50] Protective factors such as a family that values, models, and teaches empathic responding, perhaps through family volunteer projects, may mitigate the effects of video game violence. Providing prosocial video games may increase prosocial responding.[51]

CLINICS CARE POINTS

- A growing body of research indicates that exposure to violent video games contributes to desensitization to violence.
- Desensitization to violence blocks empathic responding, moral reasoning, and prosocial behavior.
- Parents should manage the media experience of children and monitor adolescent media use, limiting exposure to violent video games as much as possible.
- Parents should be counseled to discuss the differences between real and screen violence, to model and encourage nonviolent ways to solve problems, and to provide empathy-building experiences (eg, access to prosocial video games, early exposure to volunteering).
- Clinicians should evaluate the media experience of children and adolescents who are having behavioral problems.

DISCLOSURE

The author of this article have received funding from University of Toledo.

REFERENCES

1. Sypher I, Hyde LW, Peckins MK, et al. Effects of parenting and community violence on aggression-related social goals: a monozygotic twin differences study. J Abnorm Child Psychol 2019;47:1001–12.
2. Kennedy TM, Ceballo R. Emotionally numb: desensitization to community violence exposure among urban youth. Dev Psychol 2016;52:778–9.
3. Brockmyer JB. Media violence, desensitization, and psychological engagement. In: Dill K, editor. The Oxford Handbook of media psychology. New York: Oxford; 2013. p. 212–22.

4. Maibom HL. Introduction: (Almost) everything you ever wanted to know about empathy. In: Maibom HL, editor. Empathy and morality. New York: Oxford; 2014. p. 1–40.

5. Spinrad T, Eisenberg N. Empathy and morality: a developmental psychology perspective. In: Maibom HL, editor. Empathy and morality. New York: Oxford; 2014. p. 59–70.

6. Kauppinen A. At the empathetic center of our moral lives. In: Maibom HL, editor. Empathy and morality. NY: Oxford; 2014. p. 122–38.

7. Ugazio G, Majandzić J, Lamm C. Are empathy and morality linked? Insights from moral psychology, sgcial and decision neuroscience, and philosophy. In: Maibom HL, editor. Empathy and morality. New York: Oxford; 2014. p. 155–71.

8. Marsh AA. Empathy and moral deficits in psychopathy. In: Maibom HL, editor. Empathy and morality. New York: Oxford; 2014. p. 138–54.

9. Hartmann T, Krakowiak KM, Tsay-Vogel M. How violent video games communicate violence: a literature review and content analysis of moral disengagement factors. Comm Monogr 2014;81:310–32.

10. Zhao H, Juanxiang Z, Gong XX, et al. How to be aggressive from virtual to reality? Revisiting the violent video games exposure-aggression association and the mediating mechanisms. Cyberpsychol Behav Soc Netw 2021;24:56–62.

11. Hartmann T, Vorderer P. It's okay to shoot a character: moral disengagement in violent video games. J Commun 2010;60:94–119.

12. Entertainment Software Association. 2019 Essential Facts about the computer and video game industry 2021. Available at: https://www.theesa.com/essential-facts/. Accessed April 27, 2021.

13. Entertainment Software Rating Board. 2021. Available at: www.esrb.org. Accessed May 26, 2021.

14. Chivers K. 2020 video game ratings in review, and what they mean to gamers. NortonLifeLock. 2021. Available at: https://us.norton.com/internetsecurity-kids-safety-video-game-ratings.html. Accessed May 26, 2021.

15. Kaiser Family Foundation. Children and video games. Menlo Park (CA): Kaiser Family Foundation; 2002.

16. Calvert SL, Appelbaum M, Dodge K, et al. The American psychological association task force assessment of violent video games. Sci Serv Public Interest Am Psychol 2017;72(2):126–43.

17. Anderson CA, Shibuya A, Ihori N, et al. Violent video game effects on aggression, empathy, and prosocial behavior in Eastern and Western countries: a meta-analytic review. Psychol Bull 2010;136:151–73.

18. Prescott AT, Sargent JD, Hull JG. Metaanalysis of the relationship between violent video game play andphysical aggression over time. Proc Natl Acad Sci U S A 2018;115:9882–8.

19. Ferguson CJ. Do angry birds make for angry children? A meta-analysis of video game influences on children's and adolescents' aggression, mental health, prosocial behavior, and academic performance. Perspect Psychol Sci 2015;10:646–66.

20. Mathur MB, VanderWeele TJ. Finding common ground in metaanalysis "wars" on violent video games. Perspectives on Psychological Science 2019;14:705–8.

21. Funk JB, Buchman DD, Jenks J, et al. Playing violent video games, desensitization, and moral evaluation in children. J Appl Dev Psychol 2003;24:413–36.

22. Carnagey NL, Anderson CA, Bartholow BD. Media violence and social neuroscience. Curr Dir Psychol Sci 2007;16:178–82.

23. Funk JB. Children's exposure to violent video games and desensitization to violence. Child Adolesc Psychiatr Clin N Am 2005;14:387–404.
24. Funk JB, Bechtoldt H, Pasold T, et al. Violence exposure in real-life, video games, television, movies, and the internet: is there desensitization? J Adolesc 2004;27: 23–39.
25. Wei R. Effects of playing violent videogames on Chinese adolescents' proviolence attitudes, attitudes toward others, and aggressive behavior. Cyberpsychol Behav 2007;10:371–80.
26. Krahe B, Moller I. Longitudinal effects of media violence on aggression and empathy among German adolescents. J Appl Dev Psychol 2010;31:401–9.
27. Grizzard M, Tamborini R, Sherry J, et al. Repeated play reduces video games' ability to elicit guilt: evidence from a longitudinal experiment. Media Psychol 2017;20:267–90.
28. Bartholow BD, Sestir MA, Davis EB. Correlates and consequences, of exposure to video game violence: hostile personality, empathy, and aggressive behavior. Pers Soc Psychol Bull 2005;31:1573–86.
29. Breuer J, Scharkow M, Quandt T. Tunnel vision or desensitization? The effect of interactivity and frequency of use on the perception and evaluation of violence in digital games. J Media Psychol 2014;26(4):176–88.
30. DeLisi M, Vaughn MG, Gentile DA, et al. Violent video games, delinquency, and youth violence: new evidence. Youth Viol Juv Justice 2012;11:132–42.
31. Dittrick CJ, Beran TN, Mishna F, et al. Do children who bully their peers also play violent video games? A Canadian national study. J Sch Violence 2013;12: 297–318.
32. Carnagey NL, Anderson CA, Bushman BJ. The effect of video game violence on physiological desensitization to real-life violence. J Exp Soc Psychol 2007;43: 489–96.
33. Staude-Muller F, Bliesener T, Luthman S. Hostile and hardened? an experimental study on (de-)sensitization to violence and suffering through playing video games. Swiss J Psychol 2008;67:41–50.
34. Arriaga P, Adrião J, Cavaleiro FMI, et al. A "dry eye" for victims of violence: effects of playing a violent video game. Psychol Violence 2015;5(2):199–208.
35. Montag C, Weber B, Trautner P, et al. Does excessive play of violent first-person-shooter-video-games dampen brain activity in response to emotional stimuli? Biol Psychol 2012;89:107–11.
36. Perry B. Using a neurodevelopmental lens when working with children who have experienced maltreatment. Parramatta NSW (Australia): Uniting Care Children, Young People and Families; 2011. brochure.
37. Englehardt CR, Bartholow BD, Kerr GT, et al. This is your brain on violent video games: neural desensitization to violence predicts increased aggression following violent video game exposure. J Exp Soc Psychol 2011;47:1033–6.
38. Jabr MM, Denke G, Rawls E, et al. The roles of selective attention and desensitization in the association between video gameplay and aggression: an ERP investigation. Neuropsychologia 2018;112:50–7.
39. Lang PJ, Bradley MM, Cuthbert BN. International affective picture system (IAPS): affective ratings of pictures and instruction manual. Gainesville, FL: Technical Report A-8 University of Florida; 2008.
40. Goodson S, Turner KJ, Pearson SL, et al. Violent video games and the P300: no evidence to support the neural desensitization hypothesis. Cyberpsychol Behav Soc Netw 2021;24(1):48–55.

41. Gentile DA, Swing EL, Anderson CA, et al. Differential neural recruitment during violent video game play in violent and nonviolent game players. Psychol Pop Media Cult 2016;5(1):39–51.
42. Guo X, Zheng L, Wang H, et al. Exposure to violence reduces empathetic responses to other's pain. Brain Cogn 2013;82:187–91.
43. Weber R, Ritterfeld U, Mathiak K. Does playing violent video games induce aggression? Empirical evidence of a functional magnetic resonance imaging study. Media Psychol 2006;8:39–60.
44. Gao X, Pan W, Li, et al. Long-time exposure to violent video games does not show desensitization on empathy for pain: an fMRI study. Front Psychol 2017;8:650.
45. Kühna S, Kuglerb D, Schmalena K, et al. The myth of blunted gamers: no evidence for desensitization in empathy for pain after a violent video game intervention in a longitudinal fMRI study on non-gamers. Neurosignals 2018;26:22–30.
46. Regenbogen C, Herrmann M, Fehr T. The neural processing of voluntary completed, real and virtual violent and nonviolent computer game scenarios displaying predefined actions in gamers and nongamers. Soc Neurosci 2010;5: 221–40.
47. Szycik GR, Mohammadi B, Hakel M, et al. Excessive users of violent video games do not show emotional desensitization: an fMRI study. Brain Imaging Behav 2017; 11:736–43.
48. Szycik GR, Mohammadi B, Münte T, et al. Lack of evidence that neural empathic responses are blunted in excessive users of violent video games: an fMRI Study. Front Psychol 2017;8:174.
49. Funk JB. Violent video games: who's at risk?. In: Ravitch D, Viteritti J, editors. Kid stuff: marketing violence and vulgarity in the popular culture. Baltimore (MD): Johns Hopkins University Press; 2003. p. 168–92.
50. Gentile DG, Bushman BJ. Reassessing media violence effects using a risk and resilience approach to understanding aggression. Psychol Pop Media Cult 2012;1:138–51.
51. Itena GH, Boppa JA, Steiner C, et al. Does a prosocial decision in video games lead to increased prosocial real-life behavior? The impact of reward and reasoning. Comput Human Behav 2018;89:163–72.

Trauma-Focused Cognitive Behavioral Therapy for Children and Families

Judith A. Cohen, MD[a],*, Anthony P. Mannarino, PhD[b]

KEYWORDS

- Children • Adolescents • Trauma • PTSD • Parents • Families
- Trauma-focused CBT • Treatment

KEY POINTS

- Trauma-focused cognitive behavioral therapy (TF-CBT) is a family-focused treatment in which parents or caregivers (hereafter referred to as "parents") participate equally with their trauma-affected child or adolescent (hereafter referred to as "child").
- TF-CBT is a components-based and phase-based treatment that emphasizes proportionality and incorporates gradual exposure into each component.
- Parents and child receive all TF-CBT components in parallel individual sessions that allow parents and child to express their personal thoughts and feelings about the child's trauma experiences, gain skills to help the child reregulate trauma responses, and master avoidance of trauma reminders and memories.
- Families also participate in several conjoint parent-child sessions to enhance family communication about the child's trauma experiences and parental support of the child.
- Research documents that TF-CBT is effective for improving posttraumatic stress disorder and related symptoms for youth aged 3 to 18 years who experience diverse traumas and that parental participation significantly enhances the beneficial impact of TF-CBT for traumatized children.

OVERVIEW: NATURE OF THE PROBLEM

Child trauma is a serious societal problem. At least one trauma is reported by two-thirds of American children and adolescents (hereafter referred to as "children"); 33% of children experience multiple traumas before reaching adulthood.[1] Despite children's inherent resilience, trauma exposure is associated with increased risk for medical and mental health problems including posttraumatic stress disorder

[a] Department of Psychiatry, Allegheny Health Network, Drexel University College of Medicine, 4 Allegheny Center, 8th Floor, Pittsburgh, PA 15212, USA; [b] Psychiatry and Behavioral Health Institute, Allegheny Health Network, Drexel University College of Medicine, 4 Allegheny Center, Pittsburgh, PA 15212, USA
* Corresponding author.
E-mail address: judith.cohen@ahn.org

Child Adolesc Psychiatric Clin N Am 31 (2022) 133–147
https://doi.org/10.1016/j.chc.2021.05.001
1056-4993/22/© 2021 Elsevier Inc. All rights reserved.

childpsych.theclinics.com

Abbreviations	
PTSD	Posttraumatic stress disorder
TF-CBT	Trauma-focused cognitive behavioral therapy

(PTSD), depression, anxiety, substance abuse, and attempted and completed suicide.[2,3] Early identification and treatment of traumatized children can prevent these potentially serious and long-term negative outcomes.

Parents can have a significant impact on children's trauma responses. For example, lower levels of parental distress about the child's trauma and greater parental support predict more positive outcomes after child trauma exposure, whereas greater parental PTSD symptoms or lower parental support predict more negative child outcomes.[4] Involving parents in the traumatized child's treatment can effectively address these factors and thus positively affect the child's outcome.

Nonoffending parents are typically children's primary source of safety, support, and guidance. However, trauma experiences teach children that the world is dangerous and that adults may not protect them. Such children often become angry at and stop trusting their parents, leading parents to become confused and upset. Trauma-focused therapy can help parents recognize and respond appropriately to their children's trauma responses while setting appropriate behavioral limits. This approach enables parents to provide the traumatized child with ongoing opportunities to relearn (or learn for the first time) that people can be safe and trustworthy. Thus, there are many reasons to suggest that family-focused treatment that integrally includes parents significantly enhances outcomes for traumatized children. Therapists providing trauma-focused cognitive behavior therapy (TF-CBT) do not include offending parents, that is, parents who perpetrated the trauma for which the child is receiving treatment, such as a parent who perpetrated the child's sexual, physical, and emotional abuse or neglect or domestic violence. An exception is to include rejecting parents of lesbian, gay, bisexual, transgender, and queer (LGBTQ) youth (ie, parents who perpetrated emotional abuse related to the youth's sexual orientation and/or gender identity), based on strong evidence from the Family Acceptance Project (https://familyproject.sfsu.edu/) that engaging rejecting parents in family services contributes to positive outcomes for these youth.

CHILD EVALUATION OVERVIEW

Evaluating children after trauma exposure is complex and is described in detail elsewhere.[5] There are important differences between forensic and clinical evaluations, particularly after child abuse.[6] The following discussion pertains only to clinical evaluations. As with all child mental health evaluations, these evaluations should include multiple informants. At a minimum this includes interviewing the child and parent, but school reports, pediatric records, and/or other information should also be obtained as clinically indicated, and this often includes speaking to or reviewing records from the child's Child Protective Services case worker, juvenile justice parole officer, and/or past and current psychiatric treatment providers (eg, medication prescriber, in-home or wraparound services, residential treatment facility). If a forensic evaluation has been conducted by the local child advocacy center or a private evaluator, these records should also be reviewed and included in the evaluation.

To benefit from TF-CBT, children must have experienced at least one remembered trauma. The remembered trauma can be any type of trauma, including multiple traumas or complex trauma. Because avoidance is a hallmark of PTSD, children often initially minimize information about their trauma experiences and symptoms; in some cases they may completely deny having experienced trauma, thus contributing to underdiagnosis of trauma-related disorders. In addition, as noted earlier, trauma involves the betrayal of trust, typically by adults; meeting a new adult, such as a therapist, can therefore serve as a trauma reminder and lead to high levels of mistrust during the initial evaluation, particularly for children with early interpersonal trauma that involve attachment disruption.

Children should have prominent trauma-related symptoms to receive a trauma-focused treatment such as TF-CBT. A PTSD diagnosis is not necessary, although some PTSD symptoms are typically present. The use of a validated screening instrument, such as the University of California, Los Angeles PTSD Reaction Index for Diagnostic and Statistical Manual of Mental Disorders, Fifth Edition,[7] or the Children's Posttraumatic Symptom Scale for DSM-5,[8] may be useful for following these symptoms but is not a replacement for a thorough clinical interview. Evaluators must develop competence at interviewing children across the developmental spectrum for the range of trauma symptoms with which children may present. Other common diagnoses are depressive, anxiety, behavioral, or adjustment disorders. Therapists should clearly understand the manifestations of complex trauma and the multiple domains of trauma impact (ie, affective, behavioral, biological, cognitive, interpersonal, perceptual), rather than depending solely on diagnosis to determine appropriateness for trauma-focused treatment. At the same time, therapists must distinguish between complex trauma and other comorbidities. For example, children whose behavioral problems occur within a constellation of affective, biological, cognitive, and interpersonal dysregulation that is triggered by trauma reminders are likely to respond to TF-CBT and must be differentiated from children with severe primary externalizing behavior problems (eg, conduct disorder) or substance use disorders who are likely to benefit more from another evidence-based treatment that addresses these difficulties before embarking on trauma-focused treatment.

MANAGEMENT GOALS

As the description given earlier suggests, the goals of TF-CBT are to address and reregulate the individual child's domains of trauma impact, which may be summarized by, but are not limited to, the following:

(A) Affective, such as anxiety, sadness, anger, affective dysregulation
(B) Behavioral, such as avoidance of trauma reminders, self-injurious behaviors, maladaptive behaviors modeled during trauma (eg, sexual behaviors, bullying, aggression), noncompliance, severe behavioral dysregulation
(B) Biological, such as hypervigilance, poor sleep, increased startle, stomach aches, headaches, other somatic problems that interfere with functioning
(C) Cognitive/perceptual, such as intrusive trauma-related thoughts and memories, maladaptive trauma-related beliefs, dissociation, psychotic symptoms, cognitive dysregulation
(S) Social/school, such as impaired relationships with family, friends, and peers; social withdrawal; decline in school concentration, performance, and/or attendance; impaired attachment and/or trust

DESCRIPTION OF TREATMENT
Core Trauma-Focused Cognitive Behavioral Therapy Principles

Core TF-CBT principles are (1) phase-based and components-based treatment, (2) component order and proportionality of phases, (3) the use of gradual exposure in

TF-CBT, and (4) the importance of integrally including parents or other primary care-givers into TF-CBT treatment. The first 3 are briefly described here. More details about these principles are described on the authors' free Web-based training site, TF-CBT*Web* 2.0, available at www.tfcbt2.musc.edu/ and elsewhere.[9,10] The remainder of this article addresses how parents are incorporated into TF-CBT treatment.

TF-CBT is a phase-based and components-based treatment, as shown in **Box 1**.

The 3 phases of TF-CBT are stabilization, trauma narration and processing, and integration. The components of TF-CBT are summarized by the acronym PRACTICE: Psychoeducation, Parenting skills, Relaxation skills, Affect modulation skills, Cognitive coping skills, Trauma narrative and cognitive processing of the traumatic events, In vivo mastery of trauma reminders, Conjoint child-parent sessions; and Enhancing Safety. These components are described in detail later.

Fidelity to the TF-CBT model is important to ensure positive outcomes and includes the following: (1) the PRACTICE components are provided in sequential order (with some flexibility within the stabilization skills as clinically indicated and providing enhancing safety first when clinically appropriate); (2) all PRACTICE components are provided (with the exception of in vivo mastery when this is not clinically indicated); and (3) the 3 TF-CBT phases are provided in appropriate proportion and duration. For typical trauma treatment cases, TF-CBT duration is 12 to 15 sessions, and each treatment phase receives about an equal number of treatment sessions (ie, 4–5 sessions/phase). For complex trauma cases, treatment duration may be longer (16–25 sessions) and the proportionality may be altered slightly with up to half of the treatment (8–12 sessions) dedicated to stabilization skills and a quarter of the treatment (4–6 sessions) spent on trauma narrative and integration/consolidation phases, respectively, as described elsewhere.[11]

Gradual exposure is included in all of the TF-CBT components. During each session the therapist carefully calibrates and includes increasing exposure to trauma reminders while encouraging the child and parent to use TF-CBT skills in order to master negative trauma reactions evoked on exposure to these reminders. Through this process the child and parent learn new more adaptive responses. With time and ongoing practice, these responses become stronger and generalize to other situations, gradually replacing the maladaptive ones they initially had in response to the child's traumatic experience. Current evidence suggests that this may be the underlying process through which trauma-related fear is diminished.[12]

Parental Involvement in Trauma-Focused Cognitive Behavioral Therapy

Parent involvement is an integral part of the TF-CBT model, and parents receive as much time in the treatment as children. During most TF-CBT sessions, the therapist

Box 1	
Trauma-focused cognitive behavioral therapy components and phases	
Psychoeducation	Stabilization phase
Parenting skills	-
Relaxation	-
Affect modulation	-
Cognitive processing	-
Trauma narration and processing	Trauma narration phase
In vivo mastery	Integration phase
Conjoint child-parent sessions	
Enhancing safety (traumatic grief components; optional)	

spends about 30 minutes individually with the child and 30 minutes individually with the parent. Conjoint child-parent sessions are included later in the TF-CBT model to optimize open children-parent communication, both generally and related to the child's trauma experiences, as described in detail later. This structure was selected rather than family sessions based on the rationale that child trauma significantly affects parents and children and thus both benefit from individual opportunities to process personal trauma responses before meeting together to do so.

The therapist meets with the parent each session to provide the parent with each PRACTICE component as the child is receiving that component. In this manner, the parent is able to help the child to practice using the appropriate TF-CBT skills during the week when the child is not in therapy. Many parents report that the TF-CBT skills are personally helpful to them and that encouraging their children to use these is helpful in reminding the parent to use the skills as well. Often parents practice the skills together with their children at home, and this encourages the development of family resilience rituals that continue long after the end of therapy. Another reason for individual parent sessions is to facilitate open therapist-parent communication about difficult topics. For example, parents may use demeaning language to describe the child's behaviors, use ineffective discipline strategies, or say hurtful things to the child about the trauma. In such situations individual parent sessions allow the therapist to provide more appropriate parenting skills, as described later.

Most children in foster care have experienced trauma. As described later, including foster parents in treatment can enhance engagement and treatment completion for these children. In these cases, the therapist can also include the birth parent in TF-CBT if the therapist considers this to be clinically appropriate (eg, if the child is having regular visits with this parent and/or reunification is anticipated in the near future). Typically, the therapist sees the birth parent in individual sessions at a separate time from the child and foster parent and provides the birth parent with the same information as the foster parent. The therapist may consider having some sessions that include the birth and foster parents together, if clinical judgment suggests that this would be beneficial. Finally, although parental inclusion is optimal whenever possible, if there is no parent or alternative caregiver available to participate in TF-CBT treatment, youth can receive TF-CBT without parental involvement.

Orienting the Family to Trauma-Focused Cognitive Behavioral Therapy

From the beginning of treatment it is important for the therapist to help the family understand that TF-CBT is a collaborative child-parent, trauma-focused treatment. The therapist may find it useful to review the information from the child's assessment that led the therapist to conclude that trauma-focused treatment was appropriate. Collaborative child-parent treatment means that the child and parent both receive about equal time each session and that the treatment includes 2-way open communication about important issues. The parent and child may express discomfort about this (eg, lack of confidentiality in therapy). The therapist can often address this by asking each what their concerns are about sharing information and making appropriate adjustments to the extent to which this occurs when indicated. For example, youth with complex trauma who are attending TF-CBT with new foster parents often have understandable issues with trusting these new caregivers or even in trusting the therapist; the therapist needs to attend to this appropriately or the therapy may be derailed.[11]

The therapist also explains what trauma-focused treatment entails in TF-CBT, namely that (1) the therapist believes that specific problems (which the therapist describes) are related to the child's trauma experiences and (2) these problems and their relationship to the child's trauma experiences are the focus of TF-CBT and what the treatment will be addressing every session, even if other issues arise during treatment. By clarifying the nature of trauma-focused treatment, the therapist helps the family to understand what to expect and also differentiates TF-CBT from other treatments (eg, usual care) that they may have received in the past.

It is recognized that a variety of caregivers may participate in TF-CBT, and in many cases they are not the child's legal parents and/or may be a single parent or caregiver. For simplicity, the term "parents" is used throughout the following description except where specifically noted. It is important to emphasize that the therapist balances fidelity with flexibility in implementing each PRACTICE component, taking into careful consideration how best to implement the component in light of the youth's developmental level, individual interests and abilities as well as the family's culture. This is described in more detail in the TF-CBT *Web*2.0 course and elsewhere.[9,10]

STABILIZATION PHASE (4–12 SESSIONS): *PSYCHOEDUCATION*

During psychoeducation the therapist provides information about common trauma responses and trauma reminders and connects these to the child's trauma experiences and responses. The therapist also normalizes and validates these as trauma responses, because many children and parents view traumatic behavioral and affective dysregulation as the child having become a "bad kid." Helping children and parents understand these as children's trauma response, and recognizing trauma reminders that may trigger these responses, is often extremely helpful in changing the child's and parent's perspective on the problem. Importantly, this gives them hope that the child can recover and return to more positive functioning, even if the child has a long history of complex trauma and long-standing dysregulation. As with all TF-CBT components, the therapist individually tailors how to provide psychoeducation, taking into consideration the developmental level, culture, and interests of the child and family. This approach may include playing interactive psychoeducational games such as the What Do You Know game,[13] or, for teens, discussing psychoeducational information such as that available at www.nctsn.org/.

During psychoeducation for parents, the therapist provides information about the child's trauma experiences and common responses, as described earlier. Important information related to the child's trauma experience may be provided during the psychoeducation component; for example, children who have experienced sexual abuse begin to receive developmentally appropriate information about sexual abuse, including proper names for private parts. Some safety information may be incorporated during the psychoeducation component (eg, doctor's names for private body parts and information about okay and not okay touches for young children who have experienced sexual abuse). However, for children with complex trauma or those at very high risk of experiencing ongoing trauma, the enhancing safety component may be provided as the initial TF-CBT component before psychoeducation, as described in detail elsewhere.[11,14,15]

Importantly, the therapist helps children and parents begin to identify potential trauma reminders. A trauma reminder is any cue (eg, person, place, situation, sight, smell, memory, internal sensation) that remind the child of an earlier trauma; this initiates a cascade of psychological, physical, and neurobiological responses similar to those the child experienced at the time of the original trauma. When the child and parents understand this process, they can make more sense of the child's trauma responses and intervene earlier in the process to support the child's use of TF-CBT skills to interrupt, reverse, or mitigate the process. For example, a child in foster care who had experienced previous domestic violence and physical abuse from his father became angry and aggressive when yelled at by an older foster brother, leading him to hit younger children in the home. For this child, loud or angry voices were trauma reminders of his father (perpetrator), who often screamed before becoming physically abusive. The foster mother yelled at this child when he became aggressive to the younger children, causing him to become even more dysregulated. Psychoeducation about the child's trauma reminders and responses was the first step in changing this pattern.

Parenting Skills

During the parent skills component, parents gain effective strategies for responding to children's trauma-related behavioral and emotional dysregulation. The therapist typically provides specific instruction, practice, and role plays in effective parenting skills, which the therapist clinically determines according to the child's presentation and the parents' current knowledge and skills. The therapist always encourages parents to use these skills while remembering that the child's trauma-related behavioral problems occur in the context of trauma reminders. More detailed information about implementing these skills is available elsewhere.[9,10]

Time in and time out

Time out involves placing the child in a quiet place that lacks child-family interaction or other positive stimulation in order to encourage the child to reregulate his or her own emotions and/or behavior. When the larger family context is that the child has frequent positive, nurturing, and enjoyable interactions with parents (time in), the child typically finds time out to be very negative and wants to quickly return to time in. Thus, time out is most effective when the family provides high-quality time in.

Praise, positive attention, selective attention

In order to create time in, therapists instruct, practice, and role play with parents the use of praise, positive attention, and selective attention. Elements of effective praise include identifying specific behaviors the parents want the child to continue, labeling these for the child immediately after they occur, and enthusiastically praising these behaviors without taking back the praise with negative statements or qualifications.

Often parents expect, take for granted, and/or ignore children when they are behaving well and only give attention to negative or problematic behaviors. Because all children crave parental attention, this paradigm tends to reinforce children's negative behaviors, the opposite of what parents intend. In order to reverse this, positive attention requires parents to look for, attend to, and promptly provide positive attention in response to children's positive behaviors. The therapist helps parents to selectively attend to these positive behaviors while paying less attention to minor negative behaviors that, although annoying or irritating, are not dangerous (eg, pestering or intrusive behaviors, rolling eyes). By reinforcing desired behaviors with high levels of attention and not attending to undesired behaviors, parents often see marked improvements in behavioral problems.

For more significant trauma-related behavioral problems, the therapist helps the parents and child to collaboratively develop an individualized contingency reinforcement program. Such programs address specific behaviors (eg, aggression, sleep problems, sexually inappropriate behaviors), and provide specific contingencies (rewards such as stars; punishments such as loss of access to electronics) if the child does or does not meet the expectations for the number of times the behavior occurs within a given time period (typically 1 day or part of a day). Critical to the success of these programs are to (1) include the child and parents in developing the program and prizes associated with rewards; (2) choose only one behavior to address at a time rather than attempting to resolve multiple behaviors simultaneously; (3) have parents provide praise for any successes and provide contingencies and rewards promptly and consistently.

Relaxation Skills

As noted earlier, traumatized children experience multiple neurobiological changes that tend to maintain trauma responses. Parents may experience their own personal biological hyperarousal responses. Relaxation skills can help children and parents to reregulate these stress systems, both in resting states and in response to trauma reminders. The therapist provides personalized relaxation strategies to the child and encourages them to practice these on a regular basis at home. These strategies may include focused (yoga) breathing, progressive muscle relaxation, and visualization, skills that have been shown to produce physiologic relaxation responses, but therapists may also encourage children to use a variety of other relaxation strategies based on the child's own interests and developmental level. For example, young children often like to relax through blowing bubbles, dance (eg, Hokey Pokey, Chicken Song), and song (Row, Row, Row Your Boat), whereas teens often prefer to relax using their favorite music, physical activities, or crafts, such as crochet or knitting. Other children find reading or prayer relaxing. It is important for children to develop a variety of different relaxation strategies because a particular strategy (eg, exercise) may be effective in some settings (eg, after school or with peers) but not in others (eg, when going to sleep at night).

After the child has identified and practiced several acceptable relaxation strategies, the therapist meets with the parents and teaches them the relaxation skills preferred by the child. The therapist helps the parents to recognize situations in which the child may be experiencing physiologic arousal in response to trauma reminders and encourages the parents to support the child in using the relaxation skills in these situations. Parents often find relaxation skills to help with their personal anxiety or hyperarousal responses, and the therapist may encourage parents to use relaxation in this regard as well. As noted earlier, younger children may enjoy demonstrating the newly practiced relaxation skills directly to the parents in a brief joint meeting with the parents at the end of this session.

Affect Modulation Skills

During trauma experiences many children learn to not express, develop distance from, or even deny negative feelings as a self-protective mechanism. During this component the therapist helps children to become comfortable with expressing a variety of different feelings and to develop skills for managing negative affective states. These skills may include strategies such as problem solving, seeking social support, positive distraction techniques (eg, humor, journaling, helping others, perspective taking, reading, taking a walk, playing with a pet), focusing on the present, and a variety of anger management techniques. The therapist encourages the child to develop a tool kit of skills that work in different settings and for different negative feelings.[9] These skills are familiar to most child therapists; however, in contrast with other child treatments, in TF-CBT also encourages the child to implement the affective modulation skills in response to trauma reminders.

After identifying the child's preferred affective modulation strategies, the therapist then educates, practices, and role plays with the parents about how they can support the child in implementing these skills. This process often requires substantial parental tolerance and forbearance.

Helping parents to tolerate children's verbal expressions of negative emotions as a positive step toward improved affective regulation is often challenging for the therapist and parents, especially when the parents' cultural perspective views verbalizations of negative emotions (eg, using cuss words, or saying "I hate you") as disrespectful. Some parents have limited tolerance for their child's demands for parental support, especially when these come at inconvenient times or are viewed as whining or manipulative. It may be helpful for parents to practice specified TF-CBT coping skills themselves in this regard (eg, using relaxation skills to self-soothe or cognitive processing skills to modify their view of the child from "manipulative" to "needing my support" as described later).

Cognitive Processing Skills

During this component the therapist helps children recognize connections among thoughts, feelings, and behaviors (the cognitive triangle) and replace maladaptive cognitions (inaccurate or unhelpful thoughts) related to everyday events with more accurate or helpful cognitions. At this point in TF-CBT the therapist is not focusing on trauma-related thoughts with the child, because it is more effective to process these during the trauma narrative component. The therapist may use a variety of techniques to assist children with cognitive processing, including progressive logical (Socratic) questioning, responsibility pie, best friend role play, and balanced thinking (eg, replacing "either-or" with "both-and" thoughts).[9,10]

The therapist meets with the parent to introduce the cognitive triangle and begin processing the parents' maladaptive cognitions. Initially the therapist identifies parents' maladaptive cognitions related to everyday events and helps the parents use cognitive processing in this regard. Many parents have maladaptive cognitions related to the child's trauma (eg, "I should have protected my child"; "I should have known sooner that this was happening to my child"; "My child is forever damaged because of what happened"). The therapist uses clinical judgment to decide whether to begin processing the parents' trauma-related maladaptive cognitions (ie, before or during the child's trauma narrative). Additional adult cognitive processing techniques are described at CPT*Web*, available at https://www.musc.edu/cpt.

TRAUMA NARRATION AND PROCESSING PHASE (4–6 SESSIONS): *TRAUMA NARRATION AND PROCESSING*

During the trauma narration and processing phase, the therapist and child engage in an interactive process during which the child describes increasingly difficult details about personal trauma experiences, including thoughts, feelings, and body sensations that occurred during these traumas. Through this process the child describes even the most feared traumatic memories, thus "speaking the unspeakable", which enables the child to develop mastery rather than avoidance responses to these memories. Through the process of retelling these experiences, the child has multiple opportunities for repeated practice of learning mastery over traumatic memories; this also enables the child to gain perspective about trauma experiences and thereby to identify potential maladaptive cognitions that the child previously assumed to be set in stone (eg, "I deserved to be abused"). Through cognitive processing strategies learned previously the therapist helps the child to process trauma-related maladaptive cognitions. The child develops a written summary of the trauma narrative process, usually in the form of a book, poem, or song. However, it is critical to emphasize that this written narrative is only a small part of the trauma narration, which is an interactive process that occurs between the child and therapist, typically over the course of several sessions. The written narrative often is organized into chapters (eg, "About me"; "How it all began"; "Sexual abuse through the years"; "Domestic violence sucks"; Death"; "Escape"; "How I've changed"). Children who have experienced complex trauma often develop a life narrative, organized around a central trauma theme.[11] However, similar to other TF-CBT trauma narratives, these also describe specific trauma episodes in detail.

As the child meets with the therapist weekly to develop the narration, the therapist meets in parallel sessions with the parents to share the content of the child's narrative. This sharing serves multiple purposes. Few parents have heard all of the details about the child's trauma experiences, and this process allows the parents to understand the child's trauma experiences more fully. Even when the parent coexperienced the trauma, such as a mother who was the direct victim of domestic violence that the child witnessed, it is common for these perspectives to differ considerably, and a primary goal of the TF-CBT process is for nonoffending parents to hear and support the child's personal perspective. Another goal is to help parents to identify and process their personal trauma-related maladaptive cognitions; for example, hearing the child's trauma narrative may cause parents to question why their child did not tell them about the abuse sooner, and this provides an opportunity for the parents to thoroughly process this maladaptive cognition. In addition, hearing the child's trauma narrative in separate sessions with the therapist as the child is developing the narration provides the parents with adequate time to prepare for the conjoint child-parent sessions, during which the child typically shares the narrative directly with the parents. Through repeated exposure to the child's narrative the parents, as the child, gain new mastery related to hearing about their child's trauma experiences and thus more ability to model adaptive coping in the child's presence during the conjoint sessions.

INTEGRATION PHASE (4–6 SESSIONS): *IN VIVO MASTERY*

In vivo mastery is the only optional TF-CBT component. Some children develop ongoing fears and avoidance of situations that are inherently innocuous. When this avoidance significantly interferes with children's adaptive functioning, it becomes an important issue to address in treatment; TF-CBT therapists use clinical judgment to determine which children require this component. For example, a child who was sexually abused in her bedroom by a perpetrator who is no longer in the home was still afraid to sleep in her own bed, and eventually afraid to sleep at night at all, and was disrupting other family members' sleep. Another child who witnessed his sibling's sudden death at home avoided attending school for fear that his mother or another younger sibling would also die when he was not home. In vivo mastery would be appropriate for these children. In distinction to the trauma narration, which involves imaginal exposure to children's trauma experiences, in vivo (in real life) mastery involves exposure to the innocuous situation (eg, sleeping in one's own bed; returning to school) that the child fears and avoids. Through gradually facing the feared situation and learning that the feared outcome does not happen, the child learns mastery rather than avoidance.

In order to implement in vivo mastery, the therapist, child, and parents develop a fear hierarchy (sometimes referred to as a fear ladder), ascending from the least feared (1) to most feared (10) scenarios, with 10 being the desired end point (eg, the child sleeping in her own bed or attending full days of school). In vivo mastery involves gradually building up to or mastering the end point through mastering a series of smaller steps. Because in vivo mastery typically takes several weeks to complete and also because the child's adaptive functioning is significantly affected, the therapist usually begins in vivo mastery during the TF-CBT stabilization skills phase. Because relaxation and other TF-CBT stabilization skills are needed to help the child (and often the parent) to tolerate the intermediate steps in the fear hierarchy, the therapist often provides psychoeducation, parenting skills, and relaxation skills before initiating the in vivo mastery plan.

The parents are critical to the success of in vivo mastery. Children are often reluctant to surrender the fears that they believe are keeping bad things from happening, and parents provide confidence and reassurance that help the child to get through the difficult early stages of the mastery process. Parents and (if applicable) school personnel must understand why in vivo mastery is important to the child's improved adaptive functioning and must join in with the plan for it to be successful. The therapist must address the parents' concerns or fears about the child gaining mastery over the feared situation, as well as any potential secondary gain that parents may derive from the child continuing the avoidant behavior. The therapist also encourages the parents to use ongoing praise, patience, and persistence in encouraging the child to use relaxation and other TF-CBT skills during the in vivo mastery plan. These skills increasingly reap rewards for the child and parents, as the child gains increasing pride in mastering previously feared situations. If the parents do not perform the in vivo plan consistently, the child's fear and avoidance often get even worse, because of the power of intermittent reinforcement. The therapist should not embark on an in vivo plan unless the parents are fully invested in seeing the plan through to completion.

Conjoint Child-Parent Sessions

The therapist provides several conjoint child-parent sessions during the integration phase. These sessions provide opportunities for modeling and optimizing direct communication among family members about the child's traumatic experiences and other important topics before treatment closure. During conjoint sessions the therapist typically meets briefly with the parents alone (5–10 minutes) and the child alone (5–10 minutes) to prepare each for the rest of the session (conjoint child-parent session, 40–50 minutes).

The first conjoint session is usually devoted to the child sharing the trauma narrative. If this occurs, the parents have already heard and cognitively processed the child's narrative during their individual parent sessions with the therapist (described earlier). In addition to the child sharing the narrative, the child and parents may ask each other several questions that they prepared during their respective preparation time. For example, one child asked his parents "How were you feeling when I disclosed the sexual abuse"; a parent asked her son, "Did you ever blame me for your sister's death?" These questions often facilitate open discussion of deeper feelings and cognitions related to the child's trauma experiences, and many families report that these sessions were the most valuable part of their TF-CBT treatment.

Subsequent conjoint child-parent sessions may address healthy sexuality, bullying prevention, substance use refusal skills, making good peer or dating decisions, enhancing family communication, enhancing safety, or other topics according to the therapist's clinical judgment. For children who have experienced sexual abuse it is particularly important for therapists to address healthy sexuality, and parents often prefer to be included in this process. Whatever the topic the therapist selects, it is helpful to make the process fun and interactive rather than didactic. For example, most children enjoy competing with their parents in quiz or other games in which they can display their increasing knowledge and understanding about trauma and its impact. During the conjoint sessions the therapist may reintroduce What Do You Know or other therapeutic games used earlier in TF-CBT to use in this regard.

Enhancing Safety

Because traumatic experiences involve the loss of safety and betrayal of trust, it is important for children and parents to acknowledge this openly during treatment and to develop practical strategies for enhancing children's physical safety as well as emotional and interactive means for enhancing the child's internal sense of security and trust. In cases in which there is ongoing risk of trauma exposure, the enhancing safety component is provided at the beginning and often throughout TF-CBT.[11,14,15] Whether or not there is risk of repeated trauma exposure, it is usually helpful to develop a systematic family safety plan that applies to all family members, which might include no violence, no substance abuse, no secrets (ie, everyone tells and no one keeps secrets related to breaking the family safety rules), and other mutually agreed-on rules that help all family members to feel safe within the home. Communicating these to all family members and practicing their implementation at home enhance the child's belief that everyone in the family will adhere to the safety plan.

PROVIDING TRAUMA-FOCUSED COGNITIVE BEHAVIORAL THERAPY FOR SPECIFIED SETTINGS OR POPULATIONS

TF-CBT can be provided in a variety of diverse settings including residential treatment facilities, schools, foster care, inpatient, and for specified populations (eg, LGBT youth, military youth, American Indian and Alaska Native Children, Latino Children, children with developmental disabilities, youth with complex trauma, or those with ongoing trauma and/or other unsafe circumstances.) As the result of collaborative projects through the SAMHSA-funded National Child Traumatic Stress Network (www. nctsn.org/), several TF-CBT Implementation Manuals and other resources have been developed to describe details of how therapists can successfully implement TF-CBT in these settings or for these populations. These are available on the National TF-CBT Therapist Certification Web site at https://www.tfcbt.org/tf-cbt-implementation-manuals/and elsewhere.[10,11,14]

EVALUATION OF OUTCOME

TF-CBT has been evaluated in 23 randomized controlled trials in which it was compared with other active treatments/usual community care (in clinical settings) or wait-list control conditions (in refugee or war conditions). Among the currently evidence-based child trauma treatments, TF-CBT alone has been evaluated across the child and adolescent developmental spectrum (3–18 years), for multiple index trauma types (eg, sexual abuse, commercial sexual exploitation, domestic violence, disaster, war, traumatic grief, multiple and complex trauma), in different settings (eg, clinic, foster care, community domestic violence center, refugee nongovernmental organization, human immunodeficiency virus treatment centers) and in multiple countries and cultures (eg, United States, Africa, Europe, Australia, Japan) and with both mental health and nonmental health providers. In all of these studies TF-CBT has been found to be superior to the comparison conditions for improving PTSD symptoms/diagnosis, as well as other related mental health difficulties, such as depressive, anxiety, behavioral, cognitive, relationship, and other problems.

In many of these studies the impact of including parents in treatment has been examined. One study compared TF-CBT provided to child only, parent only, or child plus parent, with usual community treatment.[16] The TF-CBT conditions that included the parent led to significantly greater improvement in positive parenting practices as well as in the child's behavioral problems and child-reported depressive problems.

A study of preschoolers who had experienced sexual abuse documented that TF-CBT led to greater improvement in child outcomes as well as in parental support and parental emotional distress than nondirective supportive therapy. Improvement in parental support significantly mediated improvement in children's PTSD symptoms after treatment, and improvement in parental support and emotional distress significantly mediated improvement in children's behavioral problems at 6-month and 12-month follow-ups.[17,18] A study of children aged 8 to 14 years who experienced sexual abuse showed that TF-CBT led to significantly greater improvement in parental support, and this improvement significantly mediated improvement in children's depressive and anxiety symptoms.[19] Recent research has shown that including foster parents in TF-CBT enhanced the foster parent's engagement in treatment and the family's retention in treatment.[20,21] A community treatment study in Norway comparing TF-CBT with usual care found that, in addition to children in the TF-CBT group experiencing significantly greater improvement in PTSD, general mental health symptoms, and functional impairment,[22] parents in the TF-CBT condition experienced significantly greater improvement in their personal depressive symptoms and this mediated significantly greater improvement in children's depressive symptoms in the TF-CBT condition only.[23] Recent randomized controlled studies have documented that TF-CBT is effective for children with complex trauma and for children with traumatic grief following parental death.[24,25] Also, of particular relevance during the COVID-19 pandemic, TF-CBT also has been found to be effective when provided via telehealth in homes or school settings.[26]

SUMMARY

TF-CBT is a family-based treatment of traumatized children with strong empirical support for improving PTSD, depressive, anxiety, behavioral, cognitive, relationship, and other problems. Parents or caregivers participate in all components of TF-CBT during initial parallel individual parent sessions and later conjoint parent-child sessions. Several studies document that parental inclusion significantly contributes to positive child outcomes.

DISCLOSURE

Drs J.A. Cohen and A.P. Mannarino receive grant funding from SAMHSA (Grant No SM80056) and royalties from Guilford Press, Oxford Press, and the Medical University of South Carolina. Dr J.A. Cohen also receives royalties from Up To Date.

REFERENCES

1. Copeland W, Keeler G, Angold A, et al. Traumatic events and post-traumatic stress in childhood. Arch Gen Psychiatry 2007;64:577–84.

2. Felitti VJ, Anda RF, Nordenberg D, et al. Relationship of childhood abuse and household dysfunction to many of the leading causes of death in adults. The Adverse Childhood Experiences (ACE) Study. Am J Prev Med 1998;14(4): 245–58.

3. Kilpatrick D, Ruggiero KJ, Acierno R, et al. Violence and risk of PTSD, major depression, substance abuse/dependence and comorbidity: results for the National Survey of Adolescents. J Consult Clin Psychol 2003;71:692–700.

4. Pine DC, Cohen JA. Trauma in children: risk and treatment of psychiatric sequelae. Biol Psychiatry 2002;51:519–31.

5. Kisiel C, Conradi L, Gehernbach T, et al. Assessing the effects of trauma in children and adolescents in practice settings. Child Adolesc Psychiatr Clin N Am 2014;23:223–42.
6. Mannarino AP, Cohen JA. Treating sexually abused children and their families: identifying and avoiding professional role conflicts. Trauma Violence Abuse 2001;2:331–42.
7. Kaplow JB, Rolon-Arroyo B, Layne CM, et al. Validation of the UCLA PTSD Reaction Index for DSM-5: a developmentally informed tool for youth. J Am Acad Child Adolesc Psychiatry 2020;59(1):186–94.
8. Foa EB, Asnaai A, Aang Y, et al. Psychometrics of the child PTSD symptom Scale for DSM-5for trauma-exposed children and adolescents. J Clin Child Adolesc Psychol 2018;47(1):38–46.
9. Cohen JA, Mannarino AP, Deblinger E. Treating trauma and traumatic grief in children and adolescents. 2nd edition. New York: Guilford Press; 2017.
10. Cohen JA, Mannarino AP, Deblinger E, editors. Trauma-focused CBT for children and adolescents: treatment applications. New York: Guilford Press; 2012.
11. Cohen JA, Mannarino AP, Kleithermes M, et al. Trauma-focused cognitive behavioral therapy for youth with complex trauma. Child Abuse Negl 2012;36:528–41.
12. Craske MG, Kircanshi K, Zelikowski M, et al. Optimizing inhibitory learning during exposure therapy. Behav Res Ther 2008;46:5–27.
13. CARES Institute. What do you know? Stratford, NJ: Rowan University; 2006.
14. Cohen JA, Mannarino AP, Murray LK. Trauma-focused CBT for youth who experience ongoing traumas. Child Abuse Negl 2011;35:637–46.
15. Murray LK, Cohen JA, Mannarino AP. Trauma-focused CBT for youth who experience continuous traumatic stress. Peace Confl 2013;19:180–95.
16. Deblinger E, Lippmann J, Steer RA. Sexually abused children suffering posttraumatic stress symptoms: initial treatment outcome findings. Child Maltreat 1996;1: 310–21.
17. Cohen JA, Mannarino AP. A treatment outcome study for sexually abused preschool children: initial findings. J Am Acad Child Adolesc Psychiatry 1996;35: 42–50.
18. Cohen JA, Mannarino AP. Factors that mediate treatment outcome of sexually abused preschoolers: six and twelve month follow-ups. J Am Acad Child Adolesc Psychiatry 1998;37:44–51.
19. Cohen JA, Mannarino AP. Predictors of treatment outcome in sexually abused children. Child Abuse Negl 2000;24:983–94.
20. Dorsey S, Pullmann MD, Berliner L, et al. Engaging foster parents in treatment: a randomized trial of supplementing trauma-focused cognitive behavioral therapy with evidence-based engagement strategies. Child Abuse Negl 2014;38: 1508–20.
21. Dorsey S, Conover K, Cox JR. Improving foster parent engagement: using qualitative methods to guide tailoring of evidence-based engagement strategies. J Clin Child Adolesc Psychol 2014;43(6):877–89.
22. Jensen TK, Holt T, Ormhaug SM, et al. A randomized effectiveness study comparing trauma-focused cognitive behavioral therapy with therapy as usual for youth. J Clin Child Adolesc Psychol 2013;43:356–69.
23. Holt T, Jensen TK, Wentzel-Larsen T. The change and the mediating role of parental emotional reactions and depression in the treatment of traumatized youth: results from a randomized controlled study. Child Adolesc Psychiatry Ment Health 2014;8:11.

24. Sacher C, Keller F, Goldbeck L. Complex PTSD as proposed in ICD-11: validation of a new disorder in children and adolescents and their response to trauma-focused cognitive behavioral therapy. J Child Psychol Psychiatry 2016;58: 160–86.
25. Dorsey S, Lucid L, Martin P, et al. Task-shared trauma-focused cognitive behavioral therapy for children who experienced parental death in Kenya and Tanzania: a randomized clinical trial. JAMA Psychiatry 2020;77:464–73.
26. Stewart RW, Orengo-Aguayo R, Young J, et al. Feasibility and effectiveness of a telehealth service delivery model for treating childhood posttraumatic stress: a community-based, open pilot trial of trauma-focused cognitive behavioral therapy. J Psychother Integr 2020;30(2):274.

School-Based Interventions for Elementary School Students with Attention-Deficit/Hyperactivity Disorder

George J. DuPaul, PhD[a],*, Matthew J. Gormley, PhD[a,b],
Molly Daffner-Deming, PhD[a]

KEYWORDS

- Attention-deficit/hyperactivity disorder • Elementary school • Behavioral intervention
- Academic intervention • Self-regulation intervention
- Organizational skills intervention

KEY POINTS

- Children with attention-deficit/hyperactivity disorder experience significant behavioral, academic, and social difficulties in elementary school classrooms.
- Although stimulant and other medications can reduce symptoms, these are rarely sufficient in comprehensively addressing school functioning.
- Teachers and other school personnel can implement behavioral, academic, organizational, and self-regulation interventions to directly target symptoms and associated impairment.
- Empirical evidence supporting classroom interventions is relatively strong, particularly for behavioral treatment, organizational skills training, and self-regulation strategies.

Abbreviations	
ADHD	Attention-deficit/hyperactivity disorder
BPI	Behavioral peer intervention
CAI	Computer-assisted instruction
CWPT	Classwide peer tutoring
DRC	Daily report card
ES	
HOPS	Homework, Organization, and Planning Skills
OST	Organizational skills training
PFC	Parent friendship coaching
STP	Summer treatment program

[a] Department of Education and Human Services, Lehigh University, 111 Research Drive, Bethlehem, PA 18015, USA; [b] University of Nebraska-Lincoln, Lincoln, NE, USA
* Corresponding author.
E-mail address: gjd3@lehigh.edu

Child Adolesc Psychiatric Clin N Am 31 (2022) 149–166
https://doi.org/10.1016/j.chc.2021.08.003
1056-4993/22/© 2021 Elsevier Inc. All rights reserved.

INTRODUCTION/BACKGROUND

Children with attention-deficit/hyperactivity disorder (ADHD) frequently experience significant difficulties in school settings. This should not be surprising given that the *Diagnostic and Statistical Manual of Mental Disorders* (Fifth Edition) (*DSM-5*) criteria for this disorder require symptoms to be associated with impairment in academic and/or social functioning.[1] There are at least 3 areas that must be targeted by school-based interventions. First, the symptomatic behaviors (ie, inattention and hyperactivity/impulsivity) comprising ADHD can significantly disrupt classroom activities to a degree that deleteriously affects the learning of all children, not just those with ADHD. Thus, the reduction of disruptive, off-task behavior is an important goal for treatment. Second, symptomatic behaviors also negatively impact children's interactions with peers, teachers, and other school professionals. A common goal for school-based treatment is increased positive social interactions with concomitant reduction in verbal and physical aggression. Third, inattentive and hyperactive-impulsive behaviors frequently compromise learning and academic achievement. Thus, the success of school-based interventions is judged not only on reduction of disruptive, off-task behavior but also with respect to improvement in organizational skills and the completion and accuracy of academic work.

The need for treatment of ADHD in school settings is clear from both theoretic and empirical perspectives. From a theoretic or conceptual standpoint, it would be hard to design a more problematic setting for individuals with ADHD than the typical elementary school classroom. Students are expected to sit still, listen to academic instruction, follow multistep directions, organize their materials, keep track of homework assignments, complete independent work, wait their turn, and behave appropriately with peers and teachers. In particular, they are expected to delay responding and think before acting. These requirements are exceptionally challenging for students with ADHD given underlying difficulties in delaying their response to the environment,[2] motivation,[3] and executive functioning.[4] Thus, it is not surprising that children with ADHD experience significantly lower standardized achievement scores and school grades and higher rates of grade retention and school dropout compared with their same-aged peers.[5] In fact, one of the most ubiquitous and problematic long-term outcomes associated with ADHD is educational underachievement.[6]

The purpose of this article is to describe and review empirical evidence supporting the use of treatment strategies to address ADHD symptoms and associated impairment in elementary classroom settings. Guides to clinical decision making and collaboration with schools are provided, along with clinics care points for intervention.

INTERVENTIONS

Five broad types of intervention have been used to address symptoms and impairment exhibited by elementary school students with ADHD, including behavioral, academic, behavioral peer, organizational skills, and self-regulation strategies. Theoretic context, description, and current evidence are described separately for each intervention approach.

Behavioral Interventions

Theoretic overview
Behavioral interventions are designed to replace a socially undesirable behavior (eg, calling out) with socially appropriate equivalent (eg, raising hand before speaking). From the behavioral perspective, each behavior serves a function for the student and must be understood in the context of its antecedents (eg, teacher request) and

consequences (eg, teacher not reprimanding the student for calling out).[7] Broadly, human behavior is theorized to serve one of 4 main functions or purposes: (a) to escape or to avoid a nonpreferred activity or setting, (b) to gain attention, (c) to gain access to materials or preferred settings, or (d) for sensory stimulation.[8] Although specific behavioral interventions can vary widely depending on the target behavior, interventions typically fall into one of 2 broad categories: proactive behavioral interventions or reactive behavioral interventions. Proactive behavioral interventions target the antecedents of the problem behavior, making students less likely to engage in such behaviors (eg, reviewing classroom expectations for hand raising). Reactive behavioral interventions alter the consequences of a problem behavior by reinforcing desirable behavior (eg, praising a student for raising their hand), punishing the interfering behaviors (eg, verbal reprimand for calling out), or ignoring the problem behavior altogether (eg, not responding to the calling out but rather praising another student for raising their hand and allowing that student to provide an answer). Successful interventions are those that facilitate the function (eg, attention) of the student's interfering behavior (eg, calling out) by reinforcing a socially appropriate replacement behavior (eg, raising their hand).[9]

Description

Proactive strategies

The use of cues and prompts has been found to increase compliance with desired behavior.[10] By providing and prominently displaying positively worded developmentally appropriate, nonequivocal rules regarding classroom expectations (eg, "Raise hand and wait to be called on to speak"), teachers can improve classroom behavior.[11]

There are several basic strategies that have been found to help maintain positive classroom behavior for students with ADHD: (a) Remind students of classroom rules throughout the day and publicly praise students for appropriate behavior, (b) maintain appropriate eye contact with students, (c) remind students of behavioral expectations before the start of a new activity, (d) actively monitor students by moving throughout the classroom, (e) use nonverbal cues to redirect behavior, (f) maintain appropriate pacing for classroom activities, and (g) provide a clear schedule of activities.[9,11]

Teacher attention

Differential teacher attention has also been found effective for students with ADHD.[12] Teachers should "catch" their students being good and provide positive attention for the socially desirable behavior (eg, working quietly at their desk). Praise should occur immediately following the desired behavior and should be specific in nature (eg, "James, you're doing a great job doing your worksheet!").

In addition, teachers can extinguish minor disruptive behaviors (eg, tapping a pencil to get attention) through ignoring. It should be noted, however, that ignoring minor behaviors can sometimes lead to more intrusive behaviors (eg, calling out) because students are not gaining the attention that they desire and have not been provided a socially acceptable replacement behavior.[8] Conversely, evidence also suggests that teacher reprimands can be effective in reducing interfering behaviors.[13] Redirections should be brief, be specific in nature, occur immediately following the negative behavior, and be delivered in a neutral tone of voice.[14]

Token reinforcement/response cost

Token reinforcement provides students an immediate reinforcer (eg, sticker, plastic coin) for meeting a specific behavioral expectation (eg, fewer than 5 interruptions during a class period). These immediate reinforcers (ie, tokens) are exchanged for backup reinforcers (eg, additional computer time) later in the day or at the end of the week.[8] Token reinforcement offers flexibility, as the criteria to earn both immediate and backup reinforcers can be made increasingly stringent to help elicit longer periods or higher levels of appropriate behavior.

Response-cost systems are very similar to token reinforcement; however, within a response-cost system, students begin with access to their reward (eg, 10 minutes of computer time) and are "fined" (ie, lose points) for each occurrence of undesirable classroom behavior or interval in which behavioral expectations were not met.[8]

Although both token reinforcement and response cost have been demonstrated as effective at improving classroom behavior, their combination generally leads to greater efficacy, enhanced maintenance, and higher ratings of teacher acceptability.[15,16] In addition, the combination of response cost and token reinforcement has produced behavioral gains greater than those observed with stimulant medication within analog classroom settings.[17]

Daily report cards

Daily report cards (DRCs) are designed to improve student behavior through frequent feedback to students regarding their behavior and regular communication between school and home.[18,19] Furthermore, the DRC allows for both proactive (eg, review of behavioral expectation) and positive reactive (eg, earning reinforcers) strategies.[18] Specifically, DRCs consist of a list of clearly defined target behaviors (eg, leaves work area fewer than 3 times), a mechanism to rate the target behavior (eg, frequency, percentage, duration), across multiple periods of the day (eg, class period).[18]

Ideally, students provide the DRC to their parents, who then provide a predetermined reward (eg, screen time) if students met the behavioral requirements. This type of home-reward DRC method has been shown to be effective for students with ADHD with additional evidence suggesting programs that link school and home are more effective relative to those that are only implemented at school.[19,20] In cases whereby parents may be unable or unwilling to participate in the DRC intervention, the teacher can administer the reinforcement to the student at school as is the case for a token reinforcement or response-cost system.

Current Evidence

The empirical support for classroom behavioral interventions for elementary-students with ADHD has been well documented across single-subject research,[21] group research,[17,22] systematic reviews,[19,23] and meta-analyses.[24,25] Results of these studies have indicated that behavioral classroom management techniques meet the requirements for consideration as a well-established treatment as per recent ADHD treatment guidelines.[26]

Academic Interventions

Theoretic overview

In contrast to behavioral interventions that target ADHD symptoms, academic intervention strategies are directed at functional impairment associated with symptoms. Specifically, these interventions aim to enhance reading and math skill development as well as improved performance across all academic subject areas. Although behavioral interventions are effective in improving student attention and reducing disruptive behavior, changes to ADHD symptoms alone do not necessarily lead to concomitant gains in academic skill acquisition and achievement.[24] Furthermore, based on studies available to date, treatment approaches directed at presumed underlying cognitive deficits (eg, working memory) have not been found to significantly impact academic achievement.[27] Thus, interventions must directly target the specific academic skills that are impaired for a given student with ADHD.

Description

Interventions to address academic skill acquisition and performance difficulties associated with ADHD can include explicit instruction, computer-assisted instruction (CAI), and peer tutoring.

Explicit instruction

The most effective way to address academic underachievement is for teachers to use principles of explicit instruction when working with students. Explicit instruction is a direct approach to teaching that involves the following:

- Providing clear information to students about what is to be learned
- Instructing skills in small steps using concrete, multiple examples
- Continuously assessing student understanding
- Supporting active student participation that ensures success[28]

A critical attribute of explicit teaching is the use of instructional momentum that involves lesson pacing (eg, using a predictable lesson process that includes varied instructional activities) and managing instructional transitions (eg, giving clear directions for transitions).[29] Explicit instruction comprises 5 major components, including daily review and prerequisite skill check, teaching of new content, guided practice, independent practice, and weekly/monthly review of skill attainment.[30]

Computer-assisted instruction

From a conceptual standpoint, CAI programs have great potential to capture the attention and increase the motivation of students with ADHD.[5] Specifically, CAI programs typically include clear goals and objectives, highlight important material, simplify tasks, and provide both immediate error correction and feedback regarding accuracy, and many also use an engaging, gamelike format. Students with ADHD would presumably be more attentive to these types of teaching methods than to lectures or individual written assignments. Several controlled case studies suggest that these methods are helpful for at least some students with ADHD[31] and may be considered as an adjunct to other academic or behavioral interventions.

Peer tutoring

Similar to CAI, peer tutoring is an intervention strategy that directly addresses the needs of students with ADHD by providing immediate, frequent performance feedback and allows for active responding at the student's pace.[5] Peer tutoring involves students working in pairs and helping each other practice academic skills, typically reading, math, and spelling. The most prominent and widely studied peer tutoring program is classwide peer tutoring (CWPT[32]) in which all students are paired for tutoring with a classmate. Students are first trained in the rules and procedures for tutoring their classmates in an academic area (eg, math, spelling, reading). The tutor reads a script (eg, math problems) to the student and awards points for correct responses. The tutor corrects erroneous responses, and the student can practice the correct response for an additional point. The script (problem list) is read as many times as possible for 10 minutes, and then the students switch roles. While students are engaged in tutoring, the teacher monitors the tutoring process and provides assistance if needed. Bonus points are awarded to pairs following all the rules. At the end of the session, points are totaled, and those with the most points are declared the winners.

Current Evidence

Relative to extensive empirical support for classroom behavioral interventions, more limited evidence is available with respect to academic intervention for students with ADHD. For example, the effects of explicit instruction on academic achievement have not been specifically studied with students with ADHD; however, there is ample controlled evidence for this approach for children with emotional and behavioral disorders.[30] Furthermore, the principles underlying the explicit instruction approach have a long history of support in the behavior analytical research literature. As noted previously, several controlled case studies have demonstrated behavioral and academic improvements associated with CAI for students with ADHD.[31] More extensive evidence is available for peer tutoring. Studies have found CWPT to enhance the on-task behavior and academic performance of unmedicated students with ADHD in general education classrooms.[33] A meta-analysis of 26 single-case research design studies, including more than 900 students from the general school population (including those with and without disabilities), found moderate to large effects of peer tutoring on academic achievement.[34] Peer tutoring effects were consistently strong across dosage (ie, duration, intensity, and number of sessions), grade level, and disability status. Of particular relevance for the use of this strategy with students with ADHD, the strongest effects were found for youth with emotional and behavioral disorders relative to other disability groups. Finally, a meta-analysis of school-based intervention for ADHD studies indicated moderate to large effects of academic interventions on reading and math outcomes, primarily in the context of within-subject and single-subject design studies.[24] It is noteworthy that academic interventions were also associated with moderate effects on behavioral outcomes, suggesting that treatment targeting academic impairment may also improve ADHD symptoms.

Behavioral Peer Interventions

Theoretic overview

Youth with ADHD often struggle with peer interactions and relationships.[35] Although traditional clinic-based social skills training programs, which focus on teaching children social skills, have generally failed to reduce social impairment,[36] behavioral peer interventions (BPI) that use contingency management systems to reinforce desired social behaviors have been much more effective.

Description

In BPI, adults or peers are trained to manage contingencies in children's social situations to improve their peer relations. Perhaps the most widely researched BPI is the summer treatment program (STP), which targets children's compliance and social functioning in recreational settings, typically day camps, conducted over several weeks. Throughout daily activities, such as social skill training, coached recreational activities (eg, swimming, sports games, arts and crafts), and academic instruction, children receive continuous and intensive behavioral management from counselors (eg, activity rules, point systems, timeout, and DRCs). There are targeted positive social behaviors that youth are encouraged to display to earn points (eg, following rules, good sportsmanship, bonus points for not exhibiting negative behaviors and for answering attention questions correctly, complying with requests and commands, helping a peer, sharing with a peer, contributing positively to group, and ignoring provocation and insults) as well as specified negative behaviors, which result in lost points (eg, rule violations; poor sportsmanship, intentional and unintentional physical aggression; intention and unintentional destruction of property;

noncompliance with adult commands; stealing; interrupting, whining, or complaining; verbally abusing staff members, name calling or teasing other children, cursing lying; leaving the activity without permission).[37] Counselors record points taken or awarded to each child throughout the day, and points earned are later redeemed for privileges or rewards.

Outside of recreational settings like camp, caregivers, teachers, peers, and even siblings have also been trained to serve as social coaches and to modify contingencies to facilitate more appropriate social behavior among youth with ADHD. Regarding caregivers, the Parent Friendship Coaching (PFC) intervention instructs parents, over the course of 8 weeks, on how to encourage their child's display of socially skilled behaviors in in vivo peer interactions like play dates.[38] Sessions are manualized and aim to help parents notice their child's friendships, improve parents' communication and feedback about their child's social behavior, and train parents to teach their children friendship skills (eg, game playing, calling a peer on the phone). Similarly, teachers can pair the active teaching of classroom rules and expectations with a token reinforcement system to encourage positive social behavior and discourage negative social behavior.[39] Regarding the use of peers, interventionists can use coaching and differential attention to assist with social skill learning and practice. For example, peers can be taught to model, prompt, and reinforce social skills.[40,41] Relatedly, peers can be instructed in how to attend to or ignore their classmates' behavior to improve social functioning.[42] Last, sibling-mediated interventions can be used to reduce negative social behaviors and increase positive social behaviors. Specifically, typically developing siblings are instructed in how to prompt certain social behaviors (eg, sharing, giving help, compromising) and correctly praise their brother or sister for demonstrating that behavior.[43]

Current Evidence

Several systematic reviews of the literature have determined that BPIs are well-established treatments[19,44,45]; however, these reviews have only examined STPs and PFC. For example, results of Pelham and Fabiano[45] review suggest that STPs have medium effect sizes on displayed social behaviors with peers (d = 0.4–0.63). Relatedly, Evans and colleagues[44] cited the original pilot study of PFC that indicated small to medium effect sizes on parent reports of their child's social skills (d = 0.25–0.59).[46] Conversely, although there are individual studies examining the use of teachers, peers, and siblings as social coaches and modifiers of contingencies, there have been no systematic reviews to date that have examined the potential of these intervention agents.

Organizational Skills Interventions

Theoretic overview

Students with ADHD typically experience significant difficulties managing their time; tracking homework assignments; keeping desks, lockers, and backpacks neat and orderly; and planning long-term assignments.[5] To address these challenges, organizational skills training (OST) involves teaching and supporting students in using specific strategies, such as note-taking, organization of classroom materials, task planning, and time management.[19] As such, OST involves step-by-step instructions delivered directly to the child along with frequent, consistent opportunities for practice accompanied by clear, constructive feedback about performance. The assumption is that through scaffolded instruction, repeated practice, and consistent feedback, the student will gain organizational skills that they can use independently.

Description

Various OST programs comprise their own protocols and specific steps; however, a core set of skills and principles is shared across programs, including tracking academics-related organizational tasks, managing physical school materials, planning short- and long-term homework assignments, and effectively managing classroom and homework time. OST programs typically include a parent or teacher component wherein adults prompt and reinforce student use of organizational skills at home and in school. Parents and teachers also collect data to evaluate intervention effectiveness.

OST programs involve the following steps[47]:

1. Collect baseline data to assess pretreatment academic functioning and organizational skill level. Data can include grades on class and homework assignments, records of homework completion, and rating scales completed by teachers and parents (eg, Children's Organizational Skills Scale).[48]
2. Teach students to implement system for management of classroom materials (eg, pencils, textbooks, written assignments). Typically, this involves supporting students in using folders for different academic subjects, cleaning and organizing their binder and backpack on a regular basis, and packing materials the night before a school day.
3. Prompt students to practice skills for managing homework assignments. Students are required to write down assignments and due dates in an assignment book or enter assignments in an online homework tracking program.
4. Teach students to consistently use a system for remembering materials needed for homework completion. The system should be individualized based on student needs and interests and may include using a checklist (written or online) or reminder cards for subject-specific materials (eg, notebooks, textbooks).
5. Guide students to practice strategies for managing time to successfully complete assignments and school-related tasks. Strategies typically include writing down and monitoring assignment due dates, completing assignments in a distraction-free environment, and timing task completion to evaluate how much time to allot for future assignments.
6. Prompt students to practice planning skills for managing large, long-term assignments (eg, book reports). Students are supported in writing down due dates, breaking large assignments into subtasks (eg, smaller steps), and creating a checklist and due dates for completing subassignments.
7. Whenever possible, encourage parents and teachers to provide prompts for students to practice organizational skills and to reinforce student efforts throughout program implementation. It is vital that children are provided prompts and reinforcement at the point of performance (eg, when completing homework) in order for them to maintain strategy use over time.
8. Collect data following OST program implementation to assess whether intervention improved academic functioning and organizational skills. This involves repeating the same measures that were administered before treatment (see step 1).

Current Evidence

Several manualized OST programs are available for use with elementary school students with ADHD, including the *Organizational Skills Training for Children with ADHD*[49] and *Homework, Organization, and Planning Skills* (HOPS)[50] programs. Both programs have been evaluated in the context of randomized controlled trials involving large samples of children with ADHD. Specifically, Abikoff and colleagues[51] showed clinically significant short- and long-term improvements in children's organizational skills, homework completion, and academic progress as a function of OST relative to a wait-list control condition. In similar fashion, a randomized controlled trial of HOPS yielded significant improvements in organization and homework management relative to a wait-list control for a sample of children with ADHD.[52] These gains were maintained at 8-week follow-up and were accompanied by teacher-reported improvements in academic impairment and report card grades. Positive outcomes from these and other studies have resulted in OST being designated a well-established treatment for youth with ADHD.[19]

Self-Regulation Interventions

Theoretic overview

Self-regulation is defined as the core set of skills that enable individuals to control their behaviors, thoughts, and emotions.[53] Through self-regulation interventions, students can learn how to manage, monitor, record, and/or assess their behavior or academic performance in order to better navigate classroom expectations, engage in learning, and persist in educational tasks. Such interventions are especially important for youth with ADHD because deficits in self-control and inhibition are viewed as core features of the disorder[2] and can result in classroom difficulties, such as challenges with on-task behavior, following directions, impulse control, and task completion.

Description

Self-monitoring

One commonly used intervention technique that bolsters self-regulation skills among students with ADHD is self-monitoring. Self-monitoring is a multistage, meta-cognitive strategy in which students are taught to observe, evaluate, and record their own behavior during specific times,[54] often with the support of their teacher. Self-evaluation is embedded in the process of self-monitoring. Together, the student and the teacher can select and define the behavior to be changed as well as determine the criteria for mastery. Self-monitoring interventions are typically classified into 2 broad categories: self-monitoring of attention and self-monitoring of performance.[55] Self-monitoring of attention requires that a student be instructed to self-assess their level of attention to assigned tasks and to self-record these results when cued (eg, while doing classwork, upon hearing cue, students ask themselves, "am I on task?," and record that evaluation on a paper or digital form). The cueing is typically performed through an unobtrusive electronic device that reminds the student to self-assess (eg, beep tape that plays through headphones[56]; or vibrating timer).[57] Self-monitoring of performance requires that a student perform an academic task (eg, spelling practice) and then self-assess and record the amount of completion or accuracy of their work either during or following the task. This practice is particularly advantageous for youth with ADHD who have a tendency to make careless errors in their academic work.

Guided practice

Across self-monitoring interventions, guided practice is provided in both the desired behavior and how to complete the self-monitoring form. During the initial training phase, the teacher observes the student's target behavior and completes a self-monitoring form directed at the student's behaviors. Afterward, the student and teacher can compare forms. To strengthen self-monitoring skills and increase motivation, the teacher can provide feedback and reward the student for exhibiting targeted behaviors. Initially, this system requires greater teacher input because the student and teacher complete and compare self-monitoring forms (although checks for accuracy are not necessary to see positive behavior changes).[55] However, over time, the student should become more adept at independently managing their behavior using self-monitoring, self-evaluation, and self-reinforcement.

Mindfulness-based intervention

Another self-regulation strategy that has been become increasingly popular over the past few decades, including in schools,[58] is mindfulness-based interventions.[59] Researchers have described a 2-component model of mindfulness, which includes self-regulation of attention and attending to the present moment. Self-regulation of attention refers to bringing awareness to a point of full attention to one's thoughts, feelings, and sensations. This includes maintaining sustained attention, keeping attention flexible, focusing on current experiences, and inhibiting elaborate processing. The second component, orientation to the present moment, refers to the attitude or approach one takes in attending to the present moment and is exemplified by curiosity, openness, and acceptance.[60] A central feature of mindfulness-based interventions is teaching individuals to disengage attention from internal reactions (eg, thoughts and feelings) that elicit distress and to instead explicitly train and self-regulate attention to experiences in the present moment, without elaborative cognitive appraisals or interpretations. There are several interventions being used in schools to cultivate mindfulness, including mindfulness meditation and yoga.[61,62] These techniques teach functional skills to self-regulate attention and emotional reactivity. For meditation practices, students are typically instructed by their teacher or a video/audiorecording to focus their attention on the present moment using an anchor, such as their breath. When the mind drifts away, the focus is gently brought back to the present moment experience. Students are encouraged to try to observe their experience of the present moment without judging or modifying it. Yoga incorporates physical postures, breath control, mental concentration, and relaxation exercises that are either taught by an educator or taught by a videotape depicting an adult instructor.

Current Evidence

Numerous studies using primarily single-subject designs have examined the influence of self-regulation interventions on students diagnosed with ADHD. Regarding self-monitoring interventions, Alsalamah[63] reviewed 9 studies published between 2006 and 2016 that provided self-monitoring interventions to 24 students with ADHD (54% of whom were in elementary school). Results indicated that these strategies led to improvements in on-task behavior, increased academic performance, and decreased off-task behavior. Reid and colleagues[55] similarly conducted a meta-analysis of 16 studies published between 1974 and 2003 that evaluated self-monitoring interventions delivered to 51 students with ADHD (94% were 12 or younger). Results of this study suggested that self-monitoring interventions produced meaningful improvements for on-task behavior ($ES = 1.61$), academic productivity and accuracy ($ES = 1.32$), and reduction in inappropriate or disruptive behaviors ($ES = 1.26$). In terms of mindfulness-based interventions, the meta-analysis of Chimiklis and colleagues[61] of 11 studies examining yoga, mindfulness, and meditation interventions among 251 youth with ADHD demonstrated statistically significant effects on the following outcomes: inattention ($ES = 0.345$ as reported by parents; Hedges $g = 0.305$ as reported by teachers), hyperactivity ($ES = 0.388$ as reported by parents; Hedges $g = 0.291$ as reported by teachers), executive functioning ($ES = 0.310$), and on-task behavior ($ES = 1.219$). Relatedly, Cairncross and Miller[64] conducted a meta-analysis investigating the potential benefits of mindfulness-based interventions among individuals with ADHD, and results of their subgroup analysis focused on child-only studies ($n = 6$) demonstrated that mindfulness-based interventions significantly reduced symptoms of inattention ($d = -0.66$) and hyperactivity/impulsivity ($d = -0.47$). Despite promising results across studies, all but 2 studies[65,66] included in these meta-analyses and reviews used single-subject designs. In addition, many of the studies included in the mindfulness meta-analyses provided limited information regarding the specific nature of the intervention itself and whether medication status was held constant throughout the intervention. Thus, further research examining the how students may benefit differently from specific mindfulness techniques and the potential confounding factor of medication is needed.

CLINICAL DECISION MAKING

The extant literature does not offer strong empirical evidence indicating moderators of treatments for ADHD or contraindications and adverse effects for behavioral treatments. For example, none of the investigated child or family characteristics in the Multimodal Treatment Algorithm Study of Children with ADHD (eg, prior medication, conduct problems, anxiety, intelligence, ADHD symptom severity, public assistance, parental depression, or maternal education) were related to response to behavioral treatment.[67] The primary use of single-subject research to investigate self-regulation intervention precludes strong conclusions about moderators of treatment effect for these strategies. Still, research has indicated that initially targeting academic behaviors may be most appropriate for students with ADHD and academic difficulties, as improvements in academics may also help improve behavior.[5] Behavioral interventions may be successful in reducing symptoms of ADHD and may be implemented before, after, or in combination with medication. Some evidence suggests that medication or a combination of medication and behavioral treatment may produce the greatest reduction in ADHD symptoms,[68] although behavioral treatment alone shows comparable efficacy to medication or combination treatment among children who display significant anxiety symptoms.[69] Still, given the strong evidence for the efficacy of both medication and the behavioral, academic, OST, and self-regulatory interventions discussed in this article, considerable weight should be given to the acceptability and feasibility of potential interventions to parents and other stakeholders.

COLLABORATING WITH SCHOOLS

Given the well-documented academic, behavioral, and social difficulties experienced by children with ADHD, it is not surprising that a child's functioning at school is of primary parental concern when seeking treatment.[70] In fact, nearly one-third of children diagnosed with ADHD are first referred by school staff, second only to a parent or another family member.[71] However, interdisciplinary collaboration between schools and medical professionals is relatively limited.[72] Survey data indicate that although more than 80% of school psychologists provide psychological reports or other diagnostic information to medical professionals, only 36% provide periodic updates on student functioning, and 24% collect data regarding psychopharmacologic side effects.[73] This appears to be an underutilization of a valuable resource in treatment planning, titration, and monitoring given the shortage of child and adolescent psychiatrists[74] and the unequal distribution of child and adolescent psychiatrists across the United States.[75]

Collaboration can range from informal ad hoc relationships to formal contractual and systems-level consultative services.[76] Many tasks associated with ad hoc collaboration (eg, teacher interviews, behavioral observations) are not reimbursable via third-party payers, representing a significant barrier.[76] However, schools, and, in particular, school psychologists, are well situated to support psychopharmacologic intervention in several of the following ways: (a) Providing baseline data, (b) collecting data during a medication trial, (c) monitoring students for adverse side effects, (d) integrating psychopharmacologic interventions with academic and behavioral interventions, and (e) providing periodic progress monitoring data to prescribers to facilitate dosage increases as a child develops.[77] Furthermore, many of these evaluative procedures mirror those required of schools under the Individuals with Disabilities Education Act and/or Section 504 of the Americans with Disabilities Act. Stated differently, schools frequently have data that are necessary for a psychiatric evaluation of pediatric ADHD, or at minimum, have the skills required to obtain these data. The purpose of the following section is to highlight critical issues in collaborating with schools and school psychologists.

- There may be a need for multiple consents (ie, from the psychiatrist and the school) to be signed to meet the requirements of both HIPPA and FERPA. Parents should be informed of this requirement to both limit frustration and ensure open collaboration.
- Not all students with a *DSM-5* or *International Classification of Diseases, Ninth Revision* diagnosis of ADHD will be eligible for special education services. Special education eligibility requires evidence of adverse educational impact that is not always present among children with a medical diagnosis of ADHD.
- Conversely, most students with a medical diagnosis of ADHD *should* be eligible for some level of formal accommodations under Section 504 of the Americans with Disabilities Act.[78] These plans can include accommodations such as extra time on tests, preferential seating, and individualized behavior intervention plans, but do *not* include traditional special education services (eg, supplemental instruction in a resource room, access to a classroom aide). However, recent evidence suggests that students with ADHD may not be receiving support under Section 504.[79]
- Similar to child and adolescent psychiatrists, school psychologists face national workforce shortages resulting in large caseloads and limited time during the workday.[80] Therefore, when seeking assistance from schools, ample time should be provided to complete observations, conduct interviews, or collect rating scales.
- The use of electronic communication (eg, e-mail, patient health care portals) is likely preferable relative to attempting phone conversations during the school day. However, given the staffing shortages among both specialties, finding a mutually agreeable time can be difficult. Furthermore, even when a time can be found, school psychologists often are required to respond to student "behavior calls" to assist in deescalating a student. Such behavior calls are common[81] and can occur at unpredictable times resulting in school psychologists missing scheduled meetings during the school day.
- An initial discussion regarding the roles and responsibilities of the collaborative partners should be had at the onset of the relationship to reduce ambiguity and role confusion.[82]
- Although some school psychology training programs have created specialties within pediatric psychology that include instruction on pharmacodynamics, many do not. It has been reported that many school personnel have misconceptions about the effectiveness of medication, assuming it will be a "cure-all" for

---

Box 1
Clinics care points: Interventions for elementary school students with attention-deficit/hyperactivity disorder

Recommendations for clinicians
1. Classroom interventions should target both symptomatic behaviors and associated impairment in social and/or academic functioning.
2. Clinicians should consult with teachers and other school mental health professionals (eg, school psychologists, counselors) to support implementation of evidence-based treatment strategies.
3. Behavioral interventions have the strongest research support and include proactive strategies (eg, systematic teaching of classroom rules), teacher attention contingent on appropriate behavior, token reinforcement and response cost systems, daily report cards, and behavioral peer interventions.
4. Interventions that directly target academic skill acquisition and performance should be used, including explicit instruction, computer-assisted instruction , and peer tutoring.
5. Organizational skills training can provide direct instruction and ongoing support to enhance time management, organization of school materials, successful completion of homework, and planful engagement with long-term assignments.
6. Self-regulation strategies can supplement and extend behavioral interventions by training children to monitor, evaluate, and/or reinforce their own behavior.

---

difficult behaviors.[83] It may be helpful to describe the behavioral outcomes associated with psychotropic medications to ensure appropriate expectations.

- Relatedly, by discussing the limitations of pharmacotherapy, school psychologists can develop and implement supplemental educational, organizational, and behavioral interventions (eg, DRCs, organizational training). Evidence suggests that the integration of multiple modes of intervention can reduce the required dosage of both interventions, which can ultimately minimize side effects and maximize outcomes.[17]
- Many of the interventions described in this article are delivered in the context of in-person learning and require face-to-face interactions between students and teachers. Although remote learning is beyond the scope of this review, interventions will require adaptation when remote instruction is necessary, as was the case during the COVID-19 pandemic.

SUMMARY

Although pharmacologic treatment (primarily stimulant medication) is effective in reducing ADHD symptoms, effects are rarely sufficient in addressing the many academic and social difficulties experienced by children with ADHD.[17,67] Thus, psychosocial and educational interventions should be used not only to improve symptomatic behaviors (ie, inattention and hyperactivity/impulsivity) but also directly to address associated impairment in social and/or academic functioning (**Box 1**). Clinicians should work with teachers and school mental health professionals (eg, school psychologists, counselors) to implement behavioral, academic, OST, and/or self-regulation interventions throughout and across school years. Behavioral interventions will include some combination of proactive strategies (ie, manipulation of antecedent events), teacher attention contingent on appropriate behavior, token reinforcement and response-cost systems, DRCs, and BPIs. Academic interventions directly target achievement difficulties and involve strategies such as explicit instruction, CAI, and peer tutoring. Clinicians, school mental health professionals, or teachers can implement OST programs to enhance student time management, completion of assignments, organization of school materials, and development of plans for long-term assignments and tasks. Finally, self-regulation interventions are designed to change symptoms and associated impairment by assisting children in monitoring, evaluating, and/or reinforcing their own behavior. These interventions may be particularly helpful in weaning children off externally controlled reinforcement systems and enhancing the probability that behavior gains will generalize across settings and time. Randomized controlled trials of these school-based interventions are necessary to further explicate strategies that can be used within and across academic years to comprehensively address the many chronic and debilitating challenges students with ADHD face in elementary education settings.

DISCLOSURE

G.J. DuPaul receives author royalties from the American Psychological Association, Brookes Publishing Company, and Guilford Press for books and videos related to attention-deficit/hyperactivity disorder. M.J. Gormley and M. Daffner-Deming report no actual or potential conflicts of interest.

REFERENCES

1. American Psychiatric Association. Diagnostic and statistical manual of mental disorders. 5th edition. Washington, DC: American Psychiatric Press; 2013.
2. Barkley RA. ADHD and the nature of self-control. New York: Guilford Press; 2006.
3. Haenlein M, Caul W. Attention deficit disorder with hyperactivity: a specific hypothesis of reward dysfunction. J Am Acad Child Adolesc Psychiatry 1987;26: 356–62.
4. Brown TL. A new understanding of ADHD in children and adults: executive function impairments. New York: Routledge; 2013.
5. DuPaul GJ, Stoner G. ADHD in the schools: assessment and intervention strategies. 3rd edition. New York: Guilford; 2014.
6. Barkley RA. Attention-deficit/hyperactivity disorder: a handbook for diagnosis and treatment. 4th edition. New York: Guilford Press; 2015.
7. O'Neill R, Horner RH, Albin RW, et al. Functional assessment for problem behaviors: a practical handbook. 2nd edition. Pacific Grove (CA): Brooks/Cole; 1997.
8. Cooper JO, Heron TE, Heward WL. Applied behavior analysis. 3rd edition. Upper Saddle River (NJ): Pearson; 2020.
9. DuPaul GJ, Ervin RA. Functional assessment of behaviors related to attention-deficit/hyperactivity disorder: linking assessment to intervention design. Behav Ther 1996;27:601–22.
10. Sulzer-Azaroff B, Mayer GR. Behavior analysis for lasting change. Fort Worth (TX): Holt, Rinehart & Winston; 1991.
11. Kern L, Clemens NH. Antecedent strategies to promote appropriate classroom behavior. Psychol Sch 2007;44:65–75.
12. Pelham WE, Fabiano GA, Gnagy EM, et al. The role of summer treatment programs in the context of comprehensive treatment for attention-deficit/hyperactivity disorder. In: Hibbs ED, Jensen PS, editors. Psychosocial treatments for child and adolescent disorders: empirically based strategies for clinical practice. 2nd edition. Washington, DC: American Psychological Association; 2005. p. 377–410.
13. Pfiffner LJ, O'Leary SG. School-based psychological treatments. In: Matson JL, editor. Handbook of hyperactivity in children. Boston: Allyn & Bacon; 1993. p. 234–55.

14. Reinke WM, Herman KC, Stormont M. Classroom-level positive behavior supports in schools implementing SW-PBIS: identifying areas for enhancement. J Pos Beh Interventions 2013;15:39–50.
15. Curtis DF, Pisecco S, Hamilton RJ, et al. Teacher perceptions of classroom interventions for children with ADHD: a cross-cultural comparison of teachers in the United States and New Zealand. Sch Psychol Q 2006;21:191–6.
16. Jurbergs N, Palcic J, Kelley ML. School–home notes with and without response cost: increasing attention and academic performance in low-income children with attention-deficit/hyperactivity disorder. Sch Psychol Q 2007;22:358–79.
17. Fabiano GA, Pelham WE, Gnagy E, et al. The single and combined effects of multiple intensities of behavior modification and methylphenidate for children with attention deficit hyperactivity disorder in a classroom setting. Sch Psych Rev 2007;36:195–216.
18. Volpe RJ, Fabiano GA. Daily behavior report cards: an evidence-based system of assessment and intervention. New York: Guilford; 2013.
19. Evans SW, Owens JS, Wymbs BT, et al. Evidence-based psychosocial treatments for children and adolescents with attention-deficit/hyperactivity disorder. J Clin Child Adolesc Psychol 2018;47:157–98.
20. Vannest KJ, Davis JL, Davis CR, et al. Effective intervention for behavior with a daily behavior report card: a meta-analysis. Sch Psych Rev 2010;39:654–72.
21. Gormley MJ, DuPaul GJ. Teacher to teacher consultation: facilitating consistent and effective intervention across grade levels for students with ADHD. Psychol Sch 2015;52:124–38.
22. Gormley MJ, Sheridan SM, Dizona PJ, et al. Conjoint behavioral consultation for students exhibiting symptoms of ADHD: effects at post-treatment and one-year follow-up. Sch Ment Hea 2020;12:53–66.
23. Fabiano GA, Schatz NK, Aloe AM, et al. A systematic review of meta-analyses of psychosocial treatment for attention-deficit/hyperactivity disorder. Clin Child Fam Psychol Rev 2015;18:77–97.
24. DuPaul GJ, Eckert TL, Vilardo B. The effects of school-based interventions for attention deficit hyperactivity disorder: a meta-analysis 1996-2010. Sch Psych Rev 2012;41:387–412.
25. Iznardo M, Rogers MA, Volpe RJ, et al. The effectiveness of daily behavior report cards for children with ADHD: a meta-analysis. J Attn Dis 2020;24:1623–36.
26. Wolraich ML, Hagan JF, Allan C, et al. Clinical practice guideline for the diagnosis, evaluation, and treatment of attention-deficit/hyperactivity disorder in children and adolescents. Pediatrics 2019;144(4):e20192528.
27. Rapport MD, Orban SA, Kofler MJ, et al. Do programs designed to train working memory, other executive functions, and attention benefit children with ADHD? A meta-analytic review of cognitive, academic, and behavioral outcomes. Clin Psychol Rev 2013;33:1237–52.
28. Nelson JR, Benner GJ, Mooney P. Instructional practices for students with behavioral disorders: strategies for reading, writing, and math. New York: Guilford; 2008.
29. Rosenshine B, Stevens R. Teaching functions. In: Wittrock MC, editor. Handbook of research on teaching. 3rd edition. New York: Macmillan; 1986. p. 376–91.
30. Nelson JR, Benner GJ, Bohaty J. Addressing the academic problems and challenges of students with emotional and behavioral disorders. In: Walker HM, Gresham FM, editors. Handbook of evidence-based practices for emotional and behavioral disorders: applications in schools. New York: Guilford; 2014. p. 363–77.

31. Mautone JA, DuPaul GJ, Jitendra AK. The effects of computer-assisted instruction on the mathematics performance and classroom behavior of children with ADHD. J Atten Disord 2005;9:301–12.
32. Greenwood CR, Maheady L, Delquadri J. Classwide peer tutoring programs. In: Shinn MR, Walker HM, Stoner G, editors. Interventions for academic and behavior problems II: preventive and remedial approaches. Bethesda (MD): National Association of School Psychologists; 2002. p. 611–50.
33. DuPaul GJ, Ervin RA, Hook CL, et al. Peer tutoring for children with attention deficit hyperactivity disorder: effects on classroom behavior and academic performance. J Appl Behav Anal 1998;31:579–92.
34. Bowman-Perrott L, Davis H, Vannest K, et al. Academic benefits of peer tutoring: a meta-analytic review of single-case research. Sch Psych Rev 2013;42:39–55.
35. McQuade JD, Hoza B. Peer problems in attention deficit hyperactivity disorder: current status and future directions. Dev Disabil Res Rev 2008;14:320–4.
36. Gresham FM. Disruptive behavior disorders: evidence-based practice for assessment and intervention. New York: Guilford; 2015.
37. Pelham WE, Geriner J, Gnagy EM. Children's summer treatment program manual. Buffalo, NY: Comprehensive Treatment for Attention Disorders; 2012.
38. Mikami AY. Social skills training for youth with ADHD. In: Barkley RA, editor. Attention-deficit hyperactivity disorder: a handbook for diagnosis & treatment. 4th edition. New York: Guilford; 2015. p. 569–95.
39. DuPaul GJ, Weyand LL. School-based intervention for children with attention deficit hyperactivity disorder: effects on academic, social, and behavioural functioning. Int J Disabil Dev Educ 2006;53:161–76.
40. Plumer PJ, Stoner G. The relative effects of classwide peer tutoring and peer coaching on the positive social behaviors of children with ADHD. J Attn Disord 2005;9:290–300.
41. Vilardo BA, DuPaul GJ, Kern L, et al. Cross-age peer coaching: enhancing the peer interactions of children exhibiting symptoms of ADHD. Child Fam Bev Ther 2013;35:63–81.
42. Grauvogel-MacAleese AN, Wallace MD. Use of peer-mediated intervention in children with attention deficit hyperactivity disorder. J Appl Behav Anal 2010;43:547–51.
43. Daffner MS, DuPaul GJ, Kern L, et al. Enhancing social skills of young children with ADHD: effects of a sibling-mediated intervention. Behav Modif 2020;44:698–726.
44. Evans SW, Owen JS, Bunford N. Evidence-based psychosocial treatments for children and adolescents with attention-deficit/hyperactivity disorder. J Clin Child Adolesc Pscyh 2014;43:527–51.
45. Pelham WE, Fabiano GA. Evidence-based psychosocial treatments for attention-deficit/hyperactivity disorder. J Clin Child Adolesc Pscyh 2008;37:184–214.
46. Mikami AY, Lerner MD, Griggs MS, et al. Parental influence on children with attention-deficit/hyperactivity disorder: II. Results of a pilot intervention training parents as friendship coaches for children. J Abnorm Psychol 2010;38:737–49.
47. DuPaul, GJ, Busch, CZ, & Chunta, A. Attention-deficit/hyperactivity disorder. In: Theodore, LA, Bray M, &. Bracken, B, editors. Desk reference in school psychology. New York: Oxford University Press, in press.
48. Abikoff H, Gallagher R. The children's organizational skills scales: technical manual. North Tonawanda, NY: Multi-Health Systems; 2009.
49. Gallagher R, Abikoff HB, Spira EG. Organizational skills training for children with ADHD: an empirically supported treatment. New York: Guilford; 2014.

50. Langberg JM. Homework, organization, and planning skills (HOPS) interventions. Bethesda MD: National Association of School Psychologists; 2011.
51. Abikoff H, Gallagher R, Wells KC, et al. Remediating organizational functioning in children with ADHD: immediate and long-term effects from a randomized controlled trial. J Consult Clin Psychol 2013;81:113–28.
52. Langberg J, Epstein J, Urbanowicz C, et al. Efficacy of an organization skills intervention to improve the academic functioning of students with ADHD. Sch Psychol Q 2008;23:407–17.
53. Baumeister RF, Vohs KD. Self-regulation and the executive function of the self. J Self Ident 2003;1:197–217.
54. Nelson RO, Hayes SC. Theoretical explanations for reactivity in self-monitoring. Behav Modif 1981;5:3–14.
55. Reid R, Trout AL, Schartz M. Self-regulation interventions for children with attention deficit/hyperactivity disorder. Except Child 2005;71:361–77.
56. Rafferty LA, Arroyo J, Ginnane S, et al. Self-monitoring during spelling practice: effects on spelling accuracy and on-task behavior of three students diagnosed with attention deficit hyperactivity disorder. Behav Anal Prac 2011;4:37–45.
57. Sluiter MN, Groen Y, de Jonge P, et al. Exploring neuropsychological effects of a self-monitoring intervention for ADHD-symptoms in school. Appl Neuropsych Chil 2020;9:246–58.
58. Butzer B, Ebert M, Telles S, et al. School-based yoga programs in the United States: a survey. Adv Mind Body Med 2015;29:18–26.
59. Cullen M. Mindfulness-based interventions: an emerging phenomenon. Mind 2011;2:186–93.
60. Bishop SR, Lau M, Shapiro S, et al. Mindfulness: a proposed operational definition. Clin Psych Sci Prac 2004;11:230–41.
61. Chimiklis AL, Dahl V, Spears AP, et al. Yoga, mindfulness, and meditation interventions for youth with ADHD: systematic review and meta-analysis. J Chil Fam Stud 2018;27:3155–68.
62. Zenner C, Herrnleben-Kurz S, Walach H. Mindfulness-based interventions in schools—a systematic review and meta-analysis. Front Psych 2014;5:603.
63. Alsalamah A. Use of the self-monitoring strategy among students with attention deficit hyperactivity disorder: a systematic review. J Edu Prac 2017;8:118–25.
64. CairncrossM, Miller CJ. The effectiveness of mindfulness-based therapies for ADHD: a meta-analytic review. J Atten Disord 2020;24:627–43.
65. Abadi MS, Madgaonkar J, Venkatesan S. Effect of yoga on children with attention deficit/hyperactivity disorder. Psychol Stud 2008;53:154–9.
66. Jensen PS, Kenny DT. The effects of yoga on the attention and behavior of boys with attention-deficit/hyperactivity disorder (ADHD). J Atten Disord 2004;7:205–16.
67. Owens EB, Hinshaw SP, Kraemer HC, et al. Which treatment for whom for ADHD? Moderators of treatment response in the MTA. J Consult Clin Psychol 2003;71:540–52.
68. MTA Cooperative Group. A 14-month randomized clinical trial of treatment strategies for attention-deficit/hyperactivity disorder. Multimodal treatment study of children with ADHD. Arch Gen Psychiatry 1999;56:1073–86.
69. MTA Cooperative Group. Moderators and mediators of treatment response for children with attention-deficit/hyperactivity disorder: the multimodal treatment study of children with attention-deficit hyperactivity disorder. Arch Gen Psychiatry 1999;56:1088–96.

70. Fiks AG, Mayne S, DeBartolo E, et al. Parental preferences and goals regarding ADHD treatment. Pediatrics 2013;132(4):692–702.
71. Visser SN, Zablotsky B, Holbrook JR, et al. Diagnostic experiences of children with attention-deficit/hyperactivity disorder. National Center for Health Statistics; 2015.
72. Bradley-Klug KL, Sundman AN, Nadeau J, et al. Communication and collaboration with schools: pediatricians' perspectives. J Appl Psychol 2010;26(4):263–81.
73. Shahidullah JD, Carlson JS. Survey of nationally certified school psychologists' roles and training in psychopharmacology. Psychol Sch 2014;51(7):705–21.
74. Hunt J, Reichenberg J, Lewis AL, et al. Child and adolescent psychiatry training in the USA: current pathways. Eur Child Adolesc Psychiatry 2020;29(1):63–9.
75. Beck AJ, Page C, Buche J, et al. Estimating the distribution of the U.S. psychiatric subspecialist workforce. University of Michigan Behavioral Health Workforce Research Center; 2018. Available at: https://www.behavioralhealthworkforce. org/wp-content/uploads/2019/02/Y3-FA2-P2-Psych-Sub_Full-Report-FINAL2.19. 2019.pdf. [Accessed 15 May 2021].
76. Flaherty LT. Models of psychiatric consultation to schools. In: Weist MD, Lever NA, Bradshaw CP, et al, editors. Handbook of school mental health: research, training, practice, and policy. 2nd ed. New York, NY: Springer; 2014. p. 283–94.
77. DuPaul GJ, Carlson JS. Child psychopharmacology: how school psychologists can contribute to effective outcomes. Sch Psychol Q 2005;20(2):206–21.
78. United States Department of Education Office for Civil Rights. Dear colleague letter and resource guide on students with ADHD. 2016. Available at: https://www2. ed.gov/about/offices/list/ocr/letters/colleague-201607-504-adhd.pdf. [Accessed 15 May 2021].
79. DuPaul GJ, Chronis-Tuscano A, Danielson ML, et al. Predictors of receipt of school services in a national sample of youth with ADHD. J Attn Disord 2019; 23(11):1303–19.
80. Walcott CM, McNamara K, Hyson D, et al. Results from the NASP 2015 membership survey, part one: demographics and employment conditions. NASP Res Rep 2018;3(1):1–17.
81. Tidwell A, Flannery KB, Lewis-Palmer T. A description of elementary classroom discipline referral patterns. Preventing Sch Fail 2003;48(1):18–26.
82. Sulkowski ML, Jordan C, Nguyen ML. Current practices and future directions in psychopharmacological training and collaboration in school psychology. Sch Psychol 2009;24(3):237–44.
83. Fauenholtz S, Mendenhall AN, Moon J. Role of school employees' mental health knowledge in interdisciplinary collaborations to support the academic success of students experiencing mental health distress. Child Schools 2017;39(2):71–9.

Adolescent Eating Disorder Risk and the Social Online World: An Update

Jenna Saul, MD[a,b,*], Rachel F. Rodgers, PhD[c,d], McKenna Saul[e]

KEYWORDS

• Proeating disorder • Eating disorder • Traditional media • Social media

The role of traditional media (television and magazines) in creating eating disorder risk has long been a topic of discussion and research, but the proliferation of social media and rapid increase in the use of the Internet by adolescents generates new dynamics and new risks for the development and maintenance of eating disorders. Recent research describes the relationship between Internet and social media use and eating disorders risk, with the greatest associations found among youth with high levels of engagement and investment in photo-based activities and platforms. Here, we review different types of online content and how they are relevant to eating disorders and consider the theoretical frameworks predicting relationships between Internet and social media and eating disorders, before examining the empirical evidence for the risks posed by the online content in the development and maintenance of eating disorders. We describe proeating disorder content specifically and examine the research related to it; we then consider the implications of such content, highlight directions for future research, and discuss possible prevention and intervention strategies.

Both traditional media, notably print and television, and more contemporary forms of media, such as social media, have been identified as important sources of sociocultural appearance pressures. It has been posited that they contribute to the detrimental effects on body image and related dimensions of exposure to unrealistic and unrepresentative body types.[1] The pressure to achieve such unrealistic ideals is increased by the fact that the bodies portrayed in the media and on social media are highly unrepresentative of the general population, and accompanied by a discourse that exaggerates the extent to which body weight and shape are controllable through diet and exercise. The pressure is further exacerbated by a food environment that is not supportive of internally regulated eating patterns.[2] The reciprocal relationships between

[a] Rogers Behavioral Health, 34700 Valley Road, Oconomowoc, WI 53066, USA; [b] Child and Adolescent Psychiatry Consulting, Marshfield, WI, USA; [c] 404 INV, Department of Applied Psychology Northeastern University, 360 Huntington Avenue, Boston, MA 02115, USA; [d] Department of Psychiatric Emergency & Acute Care, Lapeyronie Hospital, CHRU Montpellier, France; [e] University of Wisconsin, Parkside, 900 Wood Road, Advising and Career Center, Kenosha, WI 53144, USA
* Corresponding author.
E-mail address: saul.jenna@gmail.com

Child Adolesc Psychiatric Clin N Am 31 (2022) 167–177
https://doi.org/10.1016/j.chc.2021.09.004
1056-4993/22/© 2021 Elsevier Inc. All rights reserved.
childpsych.theclinics.com

traditional media use, particularly print and television, and eating disorder risk have been well documented over the past 2 decades.[1] Given that contemporary youth primarily engage with nontraditional forms of media such as social media and the Internet, the association with the use of these newer forms of media and eating disorder risk warrants further exploration.[3]

The Internet is more accessible than ever, with 95% of teens owning or having access to a smartphone.[4] Indeed, 13 to 17 years old are spending more time online than ever before, with 45% endorsing that they use the Internet "almost constantly," and another 44% who report using it "several times a day." Social media platforms are also extremely popular with young people, with high percentages reporting the use of sites such as YouTube (85%), Instagram (72%), Snapchat (69%), and Facebook (51%).[4] Among adults, 18 to 29 years old are the highest Internet and social media users, with up to 84% using a social network site.[5] Frequent engagement with social media is also common among this age group, with 71% of Snapchat and 73% of Twitter users reporting daily use of the platform. In response to this increasing use, an emerging body of literature has begun to explore the relationship between Internet and social media use and eating disorder risk.

GENERAL INTERNET AND SOCIAL MEDIA USE AND EATING DISORDER RISK
Internet and Social Media in the Context of Eating Disorders

Several theoretic frameworks have been used to ground investigations of the relationship between sociocultural influences such as social media and Internet and eating disorders, including sociocultural theory, social learning theory, self-objectification theory, social identity theory, and uses and gratifications theory.[6] These theories focus on examining the ways that online and social media serve to increase the exposure to harmful appearance ideals, reinforce the centrality and importance of appearance, and model unhealthy appearance-altering behaviors and practices. Social identity theory in particular highlights how appearance and/or eating-related behaviors can be a condition for group membership, which may serve to promote eating disorders.

Online forms of media, including social media, have several attributes that make them particularly relevant to eating disorders (**Box 1**); specifically, being highly visual, targeted for specific users, highly interactive, and allowing for access to higher numbers of more specific social groups. The first attribute is their highly visual nature. The vast majority of online content is comprised of images rather than text, which

---

Box 1
Internet and Social Media Characteristics Relevant to Eating Disorders

Internet and Social Media Characteristics Relevant to Eating Disorders
- Highly visual: Little text, mostly images, with some of the most-popular applications being entirely photo-based.
- Carefully selected, curated, and editing self-presentations that emulate mainstream appearance ideals and values.
- Blurring of the distinction between commercially generated and user-generated content with intentions to increase social capital.
- Machine learning: Content tailored to each user based on previous online activity and interest. Capacity to become an increasing appearance and diet-saturated environment.
- Interactive medium that combines media influences and peer feedback.
- Capacity to bring together individuals with marginal interests and facilitate the normalization behaviors such as ED symptoms.
- Lack of moderation and supervision.
- Strong presence of commercial interests including the diet, beauty, and fitness industries.

makes it saturated in appearance-related content. Furthermore, youth may use types of social media that are particularly picture-oriented and that encourage them to spend time curating the images of themselves that appear online and examining images of their peers or celebrities. In addition, on social media, there may be a progressive blurring of the distinction between commercially generated and user-generated content. When products are presented by influencers, it may be difficult for young adolescents to identify the for-profit intent of the content. The second attribute of online media that makes it particularly relevant to eating disorders is the capacity to tailor itself to a person's interests, building on previous content views and search histories. Targeted advertising and targeted presentation of materials can lead to an online environment that becomes increasingly person-specific the more time is spent online, likened to an "echo chamber." For example, a large number of websites will have advertisements that are selectively produced based on a person's past search history; someone who has looked for dieting or weight loss-related content will be more likely to view advertisements for weight-loss products.[7] Relatedly, a content analysis of advertisements on popular websites targeting teenagers highlighted the high proportion of cosmetic and beauty products being promoted.[8] The third aspect of online media and its relevance to eating disorder is the interactive nature of the online world. Peer responses to posts, which can include teasing, are particularly salient on social media; one of the main motivations behind posting is to garner a positive response from others, often regarding appearance. An additional attribute of online media to consider as it relates to eating disorders is the opportunity for access to a wider variety of social groups than the offline world, particularly for youth. The Internet provides a space for groups with attitudes and opinions that are on the more extreme ends of the spectrum. One example of this is proeating disorder communities, which will be discussed in greater detail later in discussion.

Two of the broader characteristics of the Internet and social media that are also relevant particularly to those with eating and shape and weight concerns are the lack of oversight and moderation of Internet content, as well as its principal use for commercial purposes. One illustration of the consequences of this is the proliferation of weight loss products, apps, and other methods being sold on the Internet. Most of these products or apps are not empirically based or supported by research[9,10] and, in some cases, may even cause harm. Individuals at risk of eating disorders may not benefit from apps promoting specific behaviors such as calorie counting.

Given that the Internet and social media can theoretically be reinforcing to the development and maintenance of eating disorders, the relationship between eating disorders and Internet and social media has received increased research attention. Later in discussion, we provide a review of the empirical studies examining this relationship. Overall, the literature provides support for such a relationship with small to moderate effect sizes, depending on risk profile and type of use. It is important to remember, however, that social media use occurs in addition to exposure to traditional media and its detrimental effects on body image.

Empirical Evidence

A growing number of correlational and experimental studies, in addition to a smaller number of longitudinal studies, have provided support for the idea that there is an association between Internet use and higher levels of disordered eating behaviors and symptoms.. Earlier studies focused on examining the relationship between general Internet use and eating disorder symptoms, and provided evidence for this association in samples of adults[11,12] undergraduates,[13] and adolescents.[14–16] Furthermore, in one of the few existing longitudinal studies, Facebook use was a prospective predictor of increased eating disorder symptoms.[16] Although the directionality of these relationships remains unclear, evidence for the presence of an association is growing.

More recently, it has emerged that using photo-based online platforms, in particular social media platforms that are highly visual such as Instagram or TikTok, is most strongly related to eating disorder risk factors.[17,18] Meta-analytic findings have highlighted that while the overall magnitude of the relationship between social media use and body image outcomes was small, larger effects were found in appearance-related types of social media as well as among younger groups.[17] In addition to the use of photo-based platforms versus more general ones, the level of personal and emotional investment in their self-images has been shown to be associated with eating disorder risk. Thus, for example, among female adolescents, those who spent more time editing their images for social media reported higher levels of body dissatisfaction and dieting.[19] Similarly, among a mixed-gender group of adolescents, self-photo investment and manipulation were associated with self-reported eating disorder symptoms.[20]

Thus, involvement with photo-related activities on the Internet seems to be particularly related to eating disorder risk. Although the mechanisms accounting for this still warrant further investigation, emerging evidence points to the role of appearance comparisons.[21] In addition, feedback received from peers on social media may plan an important role. It has been shown, for example, that undergraduates who received negative feedback on their online profiles reported higher levels of eating disorder pathology.[22] However, positive feedback related to weight loss or extreme weight loss behaviors may also have harmful consequences. In addition, among adolescent girls, concerns related to peer feedback on selfies were associated with higher body image concerns and depressive symptoms.[23] Thus, concerns regarding anticipated feedback, and well as receiving negative feedback on social media, may be associated with increased eating disorder symptoms.

In sum, greater Internet and social media use, particularly photo-based applications use, had been shown to be associated with eating disorder behaviors and concerns.

HIGH-RISK GROUPS AND EATING DISORDER-SPECIFIC CONTENT

In addition to examining the relationship between Internet and social media use and eating disorder risk among youth broadly, researchers have sought to understand whether those with elevated concerns, existing eating disorders, or who are in recovery are differently affected by online and social media content. In addition, the impact of online and social media content specific to eating disorders, and how it is related to the eating disorder outcomes, has also been explored.

Higher Risk Groups

A small body of research has examined how individuals at high risk for eating disorders, or with a current or past diagnosis, may engage with or be impacted by online and social media content. For example, among young women with eating disorder symptoms in the clinical range, taking selfies but not posting them revealed an association with higher levels of eating disorder symptomatology, leading the authors to propose that such behaviors may serve as a form of body checking.[24] In addition, among young women in recovery from an eating disorder, most of whom had experienced an onset of the disorder at age 16 or younger, social media and selfie behaviors may have many layers of meaning and may be experienced in both harmful and helpful ways in the recovery process.[25]

Diet Culture-Related Content

As mentioned above, much of the content on Internet is motivated by commercial in-terests, promoting specific individuals, brands, services, or products. To date, little research has investigated how targeted advertising to individuals with existing body image and eating concerns might maintain or exacerbate eating disorder symptoms. Recent research has provided initial evidence specifically platforms and applications designed to focus on weight, eating behaviors, and exercise may indeed be unhelpful for some individuals.[26] Specifically, among college students who reported using fitness tracking applications, calorie counting, and fitness tracking were associated with eating disorder behaviors.[27] To date, however, most of this research is correla-tional such that it is unclear whether these applications cause or maintain behaviors and concerns, or whether their association with higher levels of eating disorder behav-iors is due to them being more appealing to those for whom these concerns are already in place. Similarly, little work has yet been conducted on the marketing of diet products via influencers, that is, individuals with large numbers of followers who derive financial compensation from feature products. However, the existing research shows that influencers market to children through a variety of interactive plat-forms such as TikTok or Instagram.[28] Examining how this may affect the consumption of dangerous dieting products or promote eating disorder behaviors in youth is an important area of future research.

Proeating Disorder Content

As described above, one of the ways for which the Internet is relevant to eating disor-ders is through the coming together of individuals with beliefs that only small subsets of the population hold. One such example is proeating disorder content and commu-nities that use the Internet as a means of expressing their belief in the fact that eating disorders are a life choice as opposed to a form of mental illness, and seek to support individuals in the maintenance and often concealment of their eating disorder.[29] The typical content includes pictures of very thin individuals, "thinspirations" (sometimes digitally modified so as to appear even more emaciated).[30] They also frequently pre-sent advice or "tips" for maintaining disordered eating symptomatology, including extremely unhealthy weight-loss methods or techniques for concealing symptoms from family and friends.[31] Furthermore, they often include some means of interactive communication (noticeboard, blog, or instant messaging) through which members communicate and provide each other with encouragement and support. Content an-alyses of the interactions on proeating disorder websites have highlighted the impor-tance of shared deception and concealment for fear of stigma or imposed treatment, and the way in which this reinforces the separation between the group of members and the outside world.[32] In recent years, "thinspiration" content has become more frequent on social media and has been accompanied by a newer form of content termed "fitspiration." Both of these types of content have been shown to contain mes-sages aligned with the beliefs and behaviors underlying eating disorders including the pursuit of unattainable appearance ideals, the promotion of dietary restraint and driven exercise, and the portrayal of extreme thinness.[33,34]

As might be expected, a small body of research has provided support for the asso-ciation between the use of proeating disorder websites and eating disorder symp-toms.[35,36] For example, in Schroeder[36] interviews with females undergoing eating disorder treatment, participants reported that the tips and tricks on pro-ED websites had worsened their eating disorder symptoms by prompting feelings of being "trig-gered" to act on eating disorder-related urges (eg, obsessions about nutritional information) and by teaching inappropriate, hazardous compensatory behaviors. In addition, a systematic review and meta-analysis of the findings of experimental studies investigating the effects of exposure to proeating disorder content found a consistent small to moderate size effect on eating disorder symptoms. Thus, evidence points to the fact that such websites and online content is harmful and may constitute a serious barrier to treatment.[37]

Ironically, although these proeating disorder sites focus on maintaining and promoting eating disorder symptomatology, many studies have found that a desire for social support was one of the main motivations for individuals to participate in these online communities.[29,38] Individuals suffering from eating disorders are known to experience a lack of social support in their interpersonal environment, and report shame and stigma.[27,39,40] The Internet may provide a space whereby their behaviors and attitudes will be received without judgment and whereby they can encounter others with similar experiences.

Given the evidence for the harmfulness of proeating disorder online content, efforts to limit the presence of such content have increased. Social media platforms such as Pinterest and Tumblr have banned such groups from forming, and legislation has emerged banning proeating disorder websites in Europe.[37] Professional organizations such as ANAD (Anorexia Nervosa and Associated Disorders) have been involved in advocating for the removal of proeating disorder online content despite challenges in monitoring the online space.

Regarding thinspiration and fitspiration content, a growing body of research has documented an association between viewing such content and eating disorder risk and symptoms,[41] as well as higher levels of eating disorder behaviors among those who post such content.[42] Although most of this research to date has been conducted among young adults, it is likely that these effects may also occur among younger groups.

Prorecovery Information and Support Networks

Although the Internet does allow for individuals endorsing proeating disorder positions to come together, it also facilitates the creation of support groups. Several online prorecovery groups for eating disorders do exist and have been shown to provide both information and emotional support,[43] as well as informing our understanding of the recovery process.[44] Furthermore, online groups may have flexibility in ways that face-to-face groups do not, such as being available late at night, and may fill an important gap in available resources for individuals not able to access in-person groups.[43] The creation of more supportive online content around treatment seeking is an important need, and clinicians should investigate innovative ways of using the Internet as a means of providing outreach and support.

The Internet also serves as a means of providing access to information and resources regarding eating disorders. For example, using the Internet has been shown to be a successful means of disseminating mental health first aid for eating disorders.[45] Similarly, the Reach out And Recover website provides a useful screening tool for parents or friends who are concerned about a loved one's eating behaviors. In addition, it provides a print-out summary and recommendations for referral that can be provided to a general practitioner (http://www.reachoutandrecover.com.au). Clinicians should investigate their client's use of Internet and social media, and be able to direct them and their families to accurate and helpful online resources.

RESOURCES AND FUTURE DIRECTIONS

The evidence for the ways in which the Internet and social media may serve to promote and maintain eating disorder pathology is increasing. For some individuals, it

Box 2
Social Media and Internet Use: Key findings and Practice Directions

Key Findings
- Greater Internet and social media use, particularly photo-based activities and applications, have been shown to be associated with eating disorder behaviors and risk factors.
- Individuals who are most invested in their online self-presentation, and younger adolescents, may be most vulnerable.
- Peer feedback and social comparison are emerging as important mechanisms accounting for these relationships.
- Proeating disorder websites advocate for eating disorders as a lifestyle rather than a disorder. More common "thinspiration" content also conveys harmful content promoting food rules and weight loss that are associated with eating disorders.
- Exposure to proeating disorder websites has been shown to be detrimental and increase eating disorder symptoms.
- Prorecovery content is more rare.

Practice directions & recommendations
- Clients' Internet and social media use should be taken into account as an influence for the recovery or maintenance of eating disorder symptoms.
- Clinicians should investigate innovative ways of using the Internet as a means of providing outreach and support.
- Clinicians should learn to direct clients and their families to accurate and helpful online resources.
- Clinicians should encourage clients to consider their relationship to social media, the types of content they view, and their own online contributions and activities, and in the case of minors, encourage parental mediation of online content.

may also provide a means of connecting individuals with treatment resources and helping them toward recovery. In other areas of mental health, social media markers have been used to identify those at risk for mental health concerns.[46] This is a promising approach to early identification of eating disorders, and may assist in promoting earlier access to treatment. Furthermore, increasing the number of social support resources online for individuals with eating disorders could also be a promising direction. In response to the documented effects of engagement in photo-based online activities on eating disorder risk, programs targeting media literacy around social media have started to emerge and revealed promise among adolescents.[47] More research in this direction is warranted.

More broadly, it might also be helpful for clinicians to encourage clients to consider their relationship to social media and the Internet, and their reliance on it. It has been suggested that the constant solicitations of social media might also increase stress and anxiety.[48] In the context of eating disorders, excessive use of social media may also increase the frequency of appearance comparisons and other unhelpful behaviors. Therefore, some clients may also benefit from considering the value of limiting their time online. In the case of youth, parental mediation of Internet use has been shown to be helpful and increase positive Internet use.[49] **Box 2**.

SUMMARY

The Internet and the rapid expansion of social media have created a more visual and interactive online environment, such that youth are more exposed to content promoting appearance ideals and diet culture than ever before. Social media has also given youth access to a much wider array of content and groups of people than they might otherwise encounter, in a way that can increase risk for and maintain eating disorder behaviors. Increased oversight and participation in youth's social media use by parents or other significant others who can mediate the effects of social media use, as well as education and awareness raising among adolescents as well as parents, health care professionals, and educators are sorely needed. Professional organizations have advocated for the removal of proeating disorder online content, and several sites have taken action; still, monitoring the online space is difficult. The creation of more supportive online content around treatment seeking is an important need and the effectiveness of such interventions should be measured. Clinicians should explore their patients' use of Internet and social media and consider the impact of this use on treatment. In addition, clinicians should broaden their knowledge of useful online resources that may be helpful to clients or their families.

CLINICS CARE POINTS

- Social media users who use photo-based applications such as tik-tok and Instagram, and who have a greater emotional investment with their self-image and selfie taking and editing have a higher risk for eating disorders and greater eating disorder symptoms.
- Clinicians should explore patient engagement with social media and the internet, and their reliance on it.
- Discussions about the ways that social media use may increase stress and anxiety should be explored.
- Discussions about how social media use may increase the frequency of comparisons about appearance and other behaviors that reinforce disordered eating should be explored.
- Clinicians can encourage limiting patient time online, and may engage parents to mediate use of the internet.

REFERENCES

1. Levine MP, Murnen SK. Everybody knows that mass media are/are not [pick one] a cause of eating disorders: a critical review of evidence for a causal link between media, negative body image, and disordered eating in females. J Soc Clin Psychol 2009;28(1):9–42.
2. Rodgers RF. The role of the "healthy weight" discourse in body image and eating concerns: an extension of sociocultural theory. Eat Behav 2016;22:194–8.
3. Swanson SA, Crow SJ, Le Grange D, et al. Prevalence and correlates of eating disorders in adolescents: results from the national comorbidity survey replication adolescent supplement. Arch Gen Psychiatry 2011;68(7):714–23.
4. Anderson M, Jiang J. Teens, social media & technology 2018. Pew Research Center. 2018. Available at: https://www.pewresearch.org/internet/2018/05/31/teens-social-media-technology-2018/. Accessed June 22, 2021.
5. Auxier B, Anderson M. Social media use in 2021. Pew research center. 2021. Available at: https://www.pewresearch.org/internet/2021/04/07/social-media-use-in-2021/. Accessed June 22, 2021.
6. Rodgers RF, Melioli T. The relationship between body image concerns, eating disorders and internet use, part I: a review of empirical support. Adolesc Res Rev 2016;1(2):95–119.
7. Yu J, Cude B. 'Hello, Mrs. Sarah Jones! We recommend this product!' Consumers' perceptions about personalized advertising: comparisons across advertisements delivered via three different types of media. Int J Consum Stud 2009; 33(4):503–14.
8. Slater A, Tiggemann M, Hawkins K, et al. Just one click: a content analysis of advertisements on teen web sites. J Adolesc Health 2012;50(4):339–45.

9. Pagoto S, Schneider K, Jojic M, et al. Evidence-based strategies in weight-loss mobile apps. Am J Prev Med 2013;45(5):576–82.

10. Breton ER, Fuemmeler BF, Abroms LC. Weight loss—there is an app for that! but does it adhere to evidence-informed practices? Transl Behav Med 2011;1(4): 523–9.

11. Peat CM, Von Holle A, Watson H, et al. The association between internet and television access and disordered eating in a Chinese sample. Int J Eat Disord 2015; 48(6):663–9.

12. Melioli T, Rodgers RF, Rodriges M, et al. The role of body image in the relationship between internet use and bulimic symptoms: three theoretical frameworks. Cyberpsychol Behav Soc Netw 2015;18(11):682–6.

13. Bair CE, Kelly NR, Serdar KL, et al. Does the Internet function like magazines? an exploration of image-focused media, eating pathology, and body dissatisfaction. Eat Behav 2012;13(4):398–401.

14. Tiggemann M, Slater A. NetGirls: the Internet, Facebook, and body image concern in adolescent girls. Int J Eat Disord 2013;46(6):630–3.

15. Tiggemann M, Slater A. NetTweens: the Internet and body image concerns in preteenage girls. J Early Adolesc 2014;34(5):606–20.

16. Mabe AG, Forney KJ, Keel PK. Do you "like" my photo? Facebook use maintains eating disorder risk. Int J Eat Disord 2014;47(5):516–23.

17. Saiphoo AN, Vahedi Z. A meta-analytic review of the relationship between social media use and body image disturbance. Comput Hum Behav 2019;101:259–75.

18. Holland G, Tiggemann M. A systematic review of the impact of the use of social networking sites on body image and disordered eating outcomes. Body Image 2016;17:100–10.

19. McLean SA, Paxton SJ, Wertheim EH, et al. Selfies and social media: relationships between self-image editing and photo-investment and body dissatisfaction and dietary restraint. J Eat Disord 2015;3(Suppl 1):O21.

20. Lonergan AR, Bussey K, Fardouly J, et al. Protect me from my selfie: examining the association between photo-based social media behaviors and self-reported eating disorders in adolescence. Int J Eat Disord 2020;53(5):485–96.

21. Jarman HK, Marques MD, McLean SA, et al. Social media, body satisfaction and well-being among adolescents: a mediation model of appearance-ideal internalization and comparison. Body Image 2021;36:139–48.

22. Hummel AC, Smith AR. Ask and you shall receive: desire and receipt of feedback via Facebook predicts disordered eating concerns. Int J Eat Disord 2015;48(4): 436–42.

23. Nesi J, Choukas-Bradley S, Maheux AJ, et al. Selfie appearance investment and peer feedback concern: multimethod investigation of adolescent selfie practices and adjustment. Psychol Pop Media Cult 2022. https://doi.org/10.1037/ ppm0000342. advance online publication.

24. Yellowlees R, Dingemans AE, Veldhuis J, et al. Face yourself (ie): investigating selfie-behavior in females with severe eating disorder symptoms. Comput Hum Behav 2019;101:77–83.

25. Saunders JF, Eaton AA, Aguilar S. From self (ie)-objectification to self-empowerment: the meaning of selfies on social media in eating disorder recovery. Comput Hum Behav 2020;111:106420.

26. Berry RA, Rodgers RF, Campagna J. Outperforming iBodies: a conceptual framework integrating body performance self-tracking technologies with body image and eating concerns. Sex Roles 2020;85:1–12.

27. Simpson CC, Mazzeo SE. Calorie counting and fitness tracking technology: associations with eating disorder symptomatology. Eat Behav 2017;26:89–92.

28. De Veirman M, Hudders L, Nelson MR. What is influencer marketing and how does it target children? A review and direction for future research. Front Psychol 2019;10:2685.

29. Rodgers RF, Skowron S, Chabrol H. Disordered eating and group membership among members of a pro-anorexic online community. Eur Eat Disord Rev 2012; 20(1):9–12.

30. Borzekowski DLG, Schenk S, Wilson JL, et al. e-Ana and e-Mia: a content analysis of pro–eating disorder web sites. Am J Public Health 2010;100(8):1526–34.

31. Sharpe H, Musiat P, Knapton O, et al. Pro-eating disorder websites: facts, fictions and fixes. JPMH 2011;10(1):34–44.

32. Custers K, Van den Bulck J. Viewership of pro-anorexia websites in seventh, ninth and eleventh graders. Eur Eat Disord Rev 2009;17(3):214–9.

33. Talbot CV, Gavin J, Van Steen T, et al. A content analysis of thinspiration, fitspiration, and bonespiration imagery on social media. J Eat Disord 2017;5(1):1–8.

34. Boepple L, Thompson JK. A content analytic comparison of fitspiration and thinspiration websites. Int J Eat Disord 2016;49(1):98–101.

35. Juarez L, Soto E, Pritchard ME. Drive for muscularity and drive for thinness: the impact of pro-anorexia websites. Eat Disord 2012;20(2):99–112.

36. Schroeder P. Adolescent girls in recovery for eating disorders: exploring past pro-anorexia internet community experiences. Alliant International University; 2010. Dissertation.

37. Rodgers RF, Lowy AS, Halperin DM, et al. A meta-analysis examining the influence of pro-eating disorder websites on body image and eating pathology. Eur Eat Disord Rev 2016;24(1):3–8.

38. Stewart MC, Schiavo RS, Herzog DB, et al. Stereotypes, prejudice and discrimination of women with anorexia nervosa. Eur Eat Disord Rev 2008;16(4):311–8.

39. Rouleau CR, von Ranson KM. Potential risks of pro-eating disorder websites. Clin Psychol Rev 2011;31(4):525–31.

40. Eichhorn KC. Soliciting and providing social support over the Internet: an investigation of online eating disorder support groups. J Comput Mediat Commun 2008;14(1):67–78.

41. Griffiths S, Castle D, Cunningham M, et al. How does exposure to thinspiration and fitspiration relate to symptom severity among individuals with eating disorders? Evaluation of a proposed model. Body Image 2018;27:187–95.

42. Holland G, Tiggemann M. "Strong beats skinny every time": disordered eating and compulsive exercise in women who post fitspiration on Instagram. Int J Eat Disord 2017;50(1):76–9.

43. Winzelberg A. The analysis of an electronic support group for individuals with eating disorders. Comput Hum Behav 1997;13(3):393–407.

44. Bohrer BK, Foye U, Jewell T. Recovery as a process: exploring definitions of recovery in the context of eating-disorder-related social media forums. Int J Eat Disord 2020;53(8):1219–23.

45. Melioli T, Rispal M, Hart LM, Chabrol H, Rodgers RF. French mental health first aid guidelines for eating disorders: an exploration of user characteristics and usefulness among college students. Early Interv Psychiatry 2018;12(2):229–33.

46. Shatte AB, Hutchinson DM, Fuller-Tyszkiewicz M, Teague SJ. Social media markers to identify fathers at risk of postpartum depression: a machine learning approach. Cyberpsychol Behav Soc Netw 2020;23(9):611–8.

47. McLean SA, Wertheim EH, Masters J, Paxton SJ. A pilot evaluation of a social media literacy intervention to reduce risk factors for eating disorders. Int J Eat Disord 2017;50(7):847–51.
48. Gazzaley A, Rosen LD. The distracted mind: ancient brains in a high-tech world. MIT Press; 2016.
49. Elsaesser C, Russell B, McCauley Ohannessian C, Patton D. Parenting in a digital age: a review of parents' role in preventing adolescent cyberbullying. Aggress Violent Behav 2017;35:62–72.

FURTHER READINGS

Bardone-Cone AM, Cass KM. What does viewing a pro-anorexia website do? An experimental examination of website exposure and moderating effects. Int J Eat Disord 2007;40(6):537–48.

Brotsky SR, Giles D. Inside the "pro-ana" community: A covert online participant observation. Eat Disord 2007;15(2):93–109.

Harper K, Sperry S, Thompson JK. Viewership of pro-eating disorder websites: Association with body image and eating disturbances. Int J Eat Disord 2008; 41(1):92–5.

Holland G, Tiggemann M. "Strong beats skinny every time": Disordered eating and compulsive exercise in women who post fitspiration on Instagram. Int J Eat Disord 2017;50(1):76–9.

McLean SA, Jarman HK, Rodgers RF. How do "selfies" impact adolescents' well-being and body confidence? A narrative review. Psychol Res Behav Manag 2019;12:513.

McLean SA, Wertheim EH, Masters J, Paxton SJ. A pilot evaluation of a social media literacy intervention to reduce risk factors for eating disorders. Int J Eat Disord 2017;50(7):847–51.

Norris ML, Boydell KM, Pinhas L, Katzman DK. Ana and the Internet: A review of pro-anorexia websites. Int J Eat Disord 2006;39(6):443–7.

Rodgers RF. The relationship between body image concerns, eating disorders and Internet use, part II: An integrated theoretical model. Adolesc Res Rev 2016; 1(2):121–37.

Rodgers RF, Melioli T. The relationship between body image concerns, eating disorders and internet use, part I: A review of empirical support. Adolesc Res Rev 2016;1(2):95–119.

Rodgers RF, Paxton SJ, Wertheim EH. # Take idealized bodies out of the picture: A scoping review of social media content aiming to protect and promote positive body image. Body Image 2021;38:10–36.

Rodgers RF, Skowron S, Chabrol H. Disordered eating and group membership among members of a pro-anorexic online community. Eur Eat Disord Rev 2012; 20(1):9–12.

Rodgers RF, Slater A, Gordon CS, McLean SA, Jarman HK, Paxton SJ. A biopsychosocial model of social media use and body image concerns, disordered eating, and muscle-building behaviors among adolescent girls and boys. J Youth Adolesc 2020;49(2):399–409.

Sumter SR, Vandenbosch L, Ligtenberg L. Love me Tinder: Untangling emerging adults' motivations for using the dating application Tinder. Telemat Inform. 2017;34(1):67–78.

Tiggemann M, Slater A. NetGirls: The Internet, Facebook, and body image concern in adolescent girls. Int J Eat Disord 2013;46(6):630–3.

Moving?

Make sure your subscription moves with you!

To notify us of your new address, find your **Clinics Account Number** (located on your mailing label above your name), and contact customer service at:

Email: journalscustomerservice-usa@elsevier.com

800-654-2452 (subscribers in the U.S. & Canada)
314-447-8871 (subscribers outside of the U.S. & Canada)

Fax number: 314-447-8029

Elsevier Health Sciences Division
Subscription Customer Service
3251 Riverport Lane
Maryland Heights, MO 63043

*To ensure uninterrupted delivery of your subscription, please notify us at least 4 weeks in advance of move.

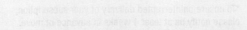